Sammy Margo has been a chartered physiotherapist for 20 years and has built up her clinic over the past 13 years. She trained as a physio at West Middlesex University Hospital and subsequently did a Masters in Physiotherapy (MSc) at University College and Middlesex Hospital. She is also the spokesperson for the Chartered Society of Physiotherapy. Sammy is a qualified Pilates and exercise instructor and incorporates this 'balanced body' approach into her treatments. She has spent many years using a practical 'hands-on' approach to the management of her clients. In addition, Sammy is actively involved in the media, including television, radio, newspaper and magazines, while still maintaining her clinical input.

THE GOOD SLEEP GUIDE

Increase your energy levels and banish
fatigue from your life forever

SAMMY MARGO,
MSc MCSP HPC MMACP AACP

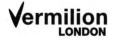

Vermilion
LONDON

1 3 5 7 9 10 8 6 4 2

Published in 2008 by Vermilion, an imprint of Ebury Publishing

Ebury Publishing is a Random House Group company

Copyright text © Sammy Margo 2008
Copyright illustrations © Victor Musson 2008

The Random House Group Limited Reg. No. 954009

Addresses for companies within the Random House Group can be found at
www.rbooks.co.uk

A CIP catalogue record for this book is available from the British Library

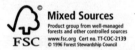

Mixed Sources
Product group from well-managed
forests and other controlled sources
www.fsc.org Cert no. TT-COC-2139
© 1996 Forest Stewardship Council

The Random House Group Limited supports The Forest Stewardship Council (FSC), the leading international forest certification organisation. All our titles that are printed on Greenpeace approved FSC certified paper carry the FSC logo. Our paper procurement policy can be found at
www.rbooks.co.uk/environment

Printed and bound in Great Britain by
Mackays of Chatham plc, Chatham, Kent

ISBN 9780091923488

Copies are available at special rates for bulk orders. Contact the sales development team on 020 7840 8487 for more information.

To buy books by your favourite authors and register for offers, visit
www.rbooks.co.uk

Contents

Acknowledgements

I am extremely grateful to all of my patients who I have been privileged to treat and who have taught me so much.

A big thank you to Gail Rebuck and my agent Ed Victor, both of whom are an inspiration to us all.

I would also like to thank Clare Hulton for her inspired creative thinking, as well as Julia Kellaway for her insight, patience and fantastic editing. Thanks to Theresa Cheung for her cutting edge research, and the rest of the team at Vermilion.

I am extremely grateful to the Chartered Society of Physiotherapy (CSP), which is working hard to 'improve the health of the nation'. For many years I have worked closely with a very special group of dedicated and forward-thinking individuals. I extend a special thanks to Prabh Salaman as well as Jennie Edmondson and Becky Darke. Thanks to the CSP for providing the illustrations and supporting this book.

A huge thanks to my work colleagues: Gayner, Dan, Karen, Steph, Julie and Tanzi who have seen me through this interesting year, as well as my parents who always encourage me to follow my dreams.

Finally a great big thank you to Simon and Isabel for letting me sleep, and Daniel my son who has yet to learn 'the art of sleep'.

Wishing you all a good night's sleep!

A Good Night's Sleep

When was the last time you had a really good night's sleep?

In my work as a physiotherapist I see many people who have problems getting a good night's sleep, but with easy techniques and a few changes to their lifestyles their problems can be resolved. If you're having problems sleeping you too can enjoy a good night's sleep, night after night, by following the practical advice in this book.

Research makes it clear that good health rests on a good night's sleep. You probably already know how important healthy eating and keeping active are for your health and wellbeing but two out of three doesn't get you there! To maximise your chances of good health and performing at your peak, both personally and professionally, you need to sleep well.

We spend more than a third of our lives asleep but sleeping well is little more than a dream for an increasing number of people. According to a recent poll conducted by the National Sleep Foundation, nearly two-thirds of adults have trouble sleeping on a few nights per week or more. In the UK recent statistics show that:

➤ 28 million workers are getting less sleep than they need for good health
➤ 63 per cent of people report at least one bad night in an average week
➤ 34 per cent regularly sleep five hours or fewer a night
➤ 18 per cent admit that they never get a really good night's sleep

This lack of shut-eye makes us more susceptible not only to poor concentration and performance at work, depleted energy levels, jaded skin and premature ageing but also to major health problems, such as high blood pressure, obesity and diabetes.

So what's keeping us awake? Back pain, stress and snoring partners are the biggest causes of poor sleeping habits but there are a number of other, less obvious, reasons why you may not be getting the quality sleep you deserve – or why you can still wake up feeling drained after eight or more hours of uninterrupted sleep.

Drawing on the very latest sleep research, and my years of experience as a physiotherapist, this book will give you sound, practical advice about how to sleep better in today's fast-paced, 24/7 world. It will cover basics from optimum sleeping positions and bedtime routines to specific situations such as dealing with jet lag or adjusting to sleeping with someone when you're used to having the bed all to yourself! There's advice, too, about what to look for when you are buying a new bed, bedclothes and pillows; what to think about when arranging your bedroom; and why recalling your dreams may be far more important for your health and wellbeing than you think.

Above all, though, the aim of this book is to show you how sleep is the magic ingredient that can make you happier, healthier, thinner and sexier. By following my practical solutions you can rest assured that a good night's sleep and waking up feeling refreshed and energised will no longer be an exception but the norm. And not only will your performance at work improve, but so too will the quality of your relationships.

WHY DO WE SLEEP?

Napoleon, Florence Nightingale and Margaret Thatcher famously got by on four hours a night. Einstein, one of history's greatest thinkers, needed eight to nine. Thomas Edison claimed it was a waste of time. So why do we sleep? This is a question that has baffled scientists for centuries, and the answer is – no one is really sure. The importance of sleep is without question. Sleep-deprivation experiments have shown that sleep is essential for concentration, clear speech, memory and hand-eye coordination. However, scientists still don't know exactly why it is so important to our survival.

Contrary to what many of us, myself included, often assume, the purpose of sleep isn't to give your body and brain a chance to recuperate from the day's activities. When you sleep you don't actually lie still and conserve energy but make frequent movements – turning over as often as 20–40 times a night and stretching continuously. And far from being 'dead to the world' during sleep, your brain is even more active than when you are awake!

Although the mystery of why we sleep has yet to be solved, one thing is clear: sleep plays a crucial role in preparing your body and mind for a productive, alert and healthy tomorrow. By making quality sleep a high priority in your life I have no doubt that you will feel healthier, happier and more productive. With increased energy and efficiency you'll find that there are more than enough hours in the day to both work and play hard.

Only when you are able to take advantage of all the restorative benefits sleep has to offer your mind and body can you discover, perhaps for the first time in years, what it feels like to be alert all day long. Follow my advice here and within a few weeks you will be able to live life as it should always be lived – to the fullest.

ONE

Why Healthy Sleep is Important

The benefits of good sleeping habits are more than just old wives' tales, they're well documented. Deep, optimal sleep has been proven to provide countless benefits to daily life – including a strengthened immune system, increased memory, a trimmer waistline and improved reaction time.

Simply put, there is just no substitute for the benefits of sleep. For anyone who wants to be healthy and successful in life, quality sleep is an essential, not a luxury. When well rested we can live our lives to the full and perform at our peak; a bad night's sleep, however, will release the demons inside us all.

TIREDNESS

Like hunger, tiredness is an entirely normal and healthy human function. Just as hunger ranges from peckish to starving, there are various degrees of tiredness:

1. Gentle weariness when yawning and a desire to lie down take over; sleep generally follows within 15 minutes of lying down.
2. More urgent tiredness; yawning may become excessive and you are asleep as soon as you hit the pillow.
3. Extreme tiredness; it is hard to keep your eyes open and you could quite literally fall asleep any time, anywhere.

The first stage of tiredness is obviously the healthy ideal, but all too often we find ourselves in the second stage or the final stage, when tiredness becomes dangerous.

THE DANGERS OF TIREDNESS

If you've ever pulled an all-nighter, you'll be familiar with the after-effects the next morning: grumpiness, grogginess, irritability and forgetfulness. Concentration is difficult and attention span almost non-existent. With continued lack of sleep, speech becomes slurred, and memory, planning and sense of time practically shut down. In fact, 17 hours of sustained wakefulness leads to a decrease in performance equivalent to a blood alcohol level of 0.05 per cent (two glasses of wine). This is the legal drink driving limit in the UK.

> 'My daily routine starts at 5am, seven days a week, when I walk the two dogs. Monday to Friday, we leave the house by 6am to drive 65 miles one way to work/school for my youngest (who sleeps for the entire trip!). Then it's work until 5pm and the drive home, those 65 miles again. Dinner, homework, bath, read, watch television, put child to bed, do the dishes, wash a load of clothes, clean up house and it's then 10pm and time to catch the last half of our favourite programme. Six hours of sleep if I'm lucky.'
> ROBIN, 41

Research shows that sleep-deprived individuals often have difficulty responding to rapidly changing situations and making rational judgements. The cost of sleep deprivation in lost production, accidents and human lives is astronomical. The National Sleep Foundation in the USA estimates that the effects of lack of sleep cost more than $100 billion a year in lost productivity. Sleep researchers believe there is enough evidence to suggest that lack of sufficient sleep is seriously affecting the UK's ability to compete in the global market.

Surgeons can make 20 per cent more mistakes after a sleepless night. This figure comes from tests using a simulator (luckily), but would the statistics for real operations be any different? It's not just scientists who are warning us: the evidence comes from doctors, police and insurance companies as well. Lack of sleep is said to contribute to two out of three road and work accidents. According to the National Highway Traffic Safety Administration in the US, each year more than 100,000 traffic accidents are caused by the effects of lack of sleep on drivers. Falling asleep at the wheel is a growing problem which accounts for one in ten of all UK road accidents. This means approximately 360 deaths and 24,000 injuries are directly attributable to sleep-related causes (Department of Transport figures).

Bear in mind that it's extreme sleep deprivation that is dangerous and not perfectly normal episodes of restlessness which everyone has from time to time. Yes, tiredness is dangerous but if someone isn't sleeping well or not getting enough shut-eye because their life is so busy, this doesn't mean they are going to make more mistakes or be involved in more accidents. What it does mean is that the quality of their sleep, and therefore their health and wellbeing, isn't as good as it should be.

BEAUTY SLEEP

Today, there are more anti-ageing products on the market than ever before, but one of the simplest and cheapest beauty treatments – helping you feel better both inside and out – is quality sleep. This is because when you sleep all the cells in your body repair and recover and human growth hormone is released; for growth hormone read 'youth hormone' (the stuff of anti-ageing supplements).

Growth hormones are rejuvenating, and when you have high levels you look and feel younger and have better skin. The best way to keep your youth hormones as high as possible is to get enough sleep. Just as drinking plenty of water is important for your skin, sleep can have a profound effect on your skin and general appearance. Several of my clients are successful models, and for them a bad night's sleep can make or break their chances of impressing on a photo-shoot the next day. It's the same with some of my elderly clients who still look great; their secret is a decent sleep routine.

Research suggests that early in the night time sleep cycle (usually between 10.30pm and 3am) people have the greatest surge of growth hormone. This period of deep sleep, or stages three and four sleep, also shows increased production and reduced breakdown of proteins; and since proteins are the building blocks needed for cell growth and repair, deep sleep may truly be beauty sleep. This suggests that going to bed before 11pm, when physiological repair is at its peak, and getting a good night's sleep could be one of the best-kept health and beauty secrets.

SLEEP AND YOUR SKIN

Besides being an essential component of a healthy lifestyle, getting six to eight hours of sleep per night helps improve the texture and the luminosity of your skin. During the night your skin is restored from the harmful effects of daily stress. That means any damage that has been done to your skin that could contribute to premature ageing is repaired. All stages of sleep are also responsible for dissolving free radicals – notorious for their contribution to early ageing.

When you do not get the sleep you need your skin suffers. The under-eye area is almost 50 per cent thinner than the skin on the rest of the face, and sleepless nights often leave behind fine lines, dark circles or puffy bags. Dark circles are caused by poor drainage of blood into the internal jugular vein. That drainage is a lot better when you're lying down than when you're standing up, so if you don't get enough shut-eye the blood tends to pool there, giving you dark half-circles. Cosmetic treatments can soften the effects of sleep deprivation but preventive medicine is the best cure.

SLEEP AND YOUR WAISTLINE

In 2007, a study published in *Sleep Medicine Reviews* revealed that the number of hours we sleep influences our risk of obesity and diabetes, and the less we sleep, the more at risk we are. Why the connection between sleep time and weight? It may all have to do with two hormones: leptin, which suppresses appetite, and ghrelin, which makes you feel hungry and is thought to play a role in long-term regulation of body weight. Sleep deprivation lowers leptin levels and raises levels of ghrelin. In addition, sleep deprivation influences our food choices, making us crave foods high in sugar and carbohydrate, which can lead to weight gain and an increased risk of insulin resistance and diabetes. All this suggests that sleep deprivation can make weight loss extremely difficult because it causes your body to work against you!

If you've got weight to lose it really is worth your while getting enough sleep. Quality sleep isn't a cure-all, and of course you have to combine it with healthy eating and regular exercise, but quality sleep may have more to do with successful weight loss and weight management than any of us ever thought possible.

Apart from the hormone shifts that occur with sleep deprivation, increasing your likelihood of gaining weight, logic would seem to suggest that:

➤ the more hours you are awake, the more hours you have to visit the fridge

➤ the less sleep you get, the more exhausted you are and the less inclined to cook properly and exercise regularly

➤ the more tired you are, the more likely you are to comfort eat

So before you blame that diet programme for your failure to lose weight, look into your sleep habits and aim for a good night's sleep.

SLEEP AND PREMATURE AGEING

'I'll sleep when I'm dead' is a phrase popular with overachievers and those who like to stay up late and rise early. However, it has now been proven that people who continue to put sleep on the back burner will in fact age at a faster pace than their counterparts who welcome sleep as a priority. Not only does lack of sleep increase the likelihood of wrinkles by preventing growth hormone from rejuvenating and repairing skin, it has also been shown to result in higher stress hormone levels. Stress hormones like cortisol lower your immunity, leaving you vulnerable to diseases such as high blood pressure and diabetes that cause early ageing.

Studies have also shown that those who sleep for six to eight hours a night actually live longer than people who sleep for less than four hours or more than eight hours, making the right amount of quality sleep one of the best anti-ageing treatments out there.

SLEEP AND MOOD

'Sleep is for wimps,' Margaret Thatcher famously said, and workers who burn the midnight oil seem to agree. Psychologists and various health experts beg to differ. Increasingly, they see sleep deprivation in its various forms as the underlying cause of stress-related physical and mental illness, and they insist that six to eight hours' sleep a night is essential for emotional well-being. My experience as a physiotherapist has led me to the same conclusion.

> *Jonathan, 44, a well-liked CEO of a successful company, was happy with his success. However, his more ambitious business partner was keen to expand and pushed hard for this to happen. The company grew rapidly but Jonathan found it hard to adjust to the new momentum. He started to have problems sleeping because his mind couldn't switch off. He tried drinking alcohol at night, which helped initially but led to a worsening sleep pattern that made him even more tired. He also loaded up on caffeine during the day to stay awake. In a matter of months he had changed from a considerate, approachable employer to an irritable, impatient and easily annoyed boss.*

Studies confirm that there is a close relationship between depression and sleep deprivation. This is because activity in parts of the brain that control emotions, decision-making processes and social interactions is drastically reduced during deep sleep, suggesting that quality sleep may help people maintain optimal emotional and social functioning while they are awake. So yet another benefit of sleep is that it can help us not only look good but also feel good, have better relationships, win friends and influence people.

SLEEP ON IT

The age-old advice to 'sleep on it' could well be true. Studies show that people given a mathematical problem before they go to bed have higher chances of solving it the next morning. This is because memory consolidation happens during sleep. Anything you read just before going to bed is more likely to be encoded as a long-term memory. So if you're studying for an exam, preparing for a presentation or have a problem to solve, reviewing the material half an hour before you turn the lights off can help you come up with a solution the next day.

TIME TO PUT SLEEP FIRST

How many more reasons do we need before we realise the benefits of sleep and the importance of sleep in our lives? And yet, still we skimp, putting everything else in our lives first. Four hours' sleep, five hours' sleep, but anything less than we need is asking for trouble. If a healthy sleep pattern isn't established it could lead to poor memory and coordination, and possibly to weight gain, mood swings and wrinkles.

Sleep isn't a cure-all, and too much sleep isn't healthy either. However, the right amount of sleep can profoundly affect your health, mood and productivity, proving that things really do look and feel better in the morning.

There is no hard-and-fast rule regarding the right amount of sleep. Much will depend on your age, build and personal circumstances. For example, if you are running a marathon or are going through a stressful divorce you may need much more sleep than usual. The key is to find the amount of sleep that is right for you and just you.

* * *

Enough pillow talk! It's clear that a quality night's sleep is absolutely essential for performing at your peak and for feeling and looking good. It's also clear that episodes of restlessness, which we all have from time to time, are not going to kill you; it's chronic and long-term sleep deprivation that is dangerous. What is needed is a sensible but flexible healthy sleep plan designed for people with busy lives. And this book will help you design such a plan.

TWO

Understanding Sleep

Considering that we spend up to a third of our lives asleep, it's remarkable that very little was known about sleep until fairly recently. Understanding why we tend to fall asleep or stay awake at particular times, and the consequences of not getting enough sleep, can help us discover how much sleep we need to feel fully alert, energetic and ready to perform at our peak.

THE NIGHTLY SLEEP CYCLE

Many people think that as soon as we go to bed we fall into a deep sleep and then move into lighter sleep before waking but this isn't what actually happens. Sleep, a stage beyond closing the eyes, can be divided into several stages of light and deep sleep. Each recurring cycle lasts 90–110 minutes and is divided into two stages: non-REM (which is split into four further stages) and REM sleep.

NON-REM SLEEP

Stage 1: Light Sleep

During the first stage of sleep, we're half-awake and half-asleep. Our muscle activity slows down and slight twitching can occur. This period of light sleep may last only a few minutes, meaning we can be woken easily and occupies approximately 2–5 per cent of a normal night of sleep.

Stage 2: Light–Intermediate Sleep

Within 10 minutes of light sleep, we enter the second stage, which initially lasts for around 20 minutes. The breathing pattern and heart rate start to slow down. This period accounts for the largest part of human sleep (45–55 per cent).

Stages 3 and 4: Deep Sleep

During the third stage, the brain begins to produce delta waves. These are large (high amplitude) and slow (low frequency). Breathing and heart rate are at their lowest levels.

The fourth stage is characterised by rhythmic breathing and limited muscle activity and comprises 40 per cent of a normal night of sleep. If we are woken during deep sleep we do not adjust immediately and often feel groggy and dis-oriented for several minutes.

REM SLEEP

The first rapid eye movement (REM) period usually begins about 70–90 minutes after we fall into deep sleep. We have around three to five REM episodes a night. Although we are not conscious, the brain is very active, often more so than when we are awake. This is the period when most dreams occur. Our eyes dart around (hence the name REM for rapid eye movement), and our breathing rate and blood pressure rise. However, our bodies are effectively paralysed, which is thought to be nature's way of preventing us from acting out our dreams. After REM sleep, the whole cycle begins again.

It seems that sleeping is an active and dynamic, rather than passive, state. Research has made it clear that the various stages of sleep we experience every night are delineated by a level of brain activity that is sometimes more active than when the brain is 'awake'. We know that the 'sleeping' brain plays an important part in boosting immunity, regulating cardiovascular function, energising the body and preparing the mind for peak performance. And, according to the very latest research, even the dreams we have during sleep may be meaningful (*see Chapter 16*).

CIRCADIAN RHYTHMS

The reason why we fall asleep or stay awake at particular times during the day and night depends on daily cycles of sleep and wakefulness called circadian rhythms.

Circadian rhythms are regular changes in mental and physical characteristics that occur in the course of a day (circadian is Latin for 'around a day'). Most circadian rhythms are controlled by the body's biological clock. This clock, called the suprachiasmatic nucleus, or SCN, is actually a pair of pinhead-sized brain structures that together contain about 20,000 neurons. The SCN rests in a part of the brain called the hypothalamus, just above the point where the optic nerves cross.

Signals from the SCN travel to several brain regions, including the pineal gland, which responds to light-induced signals by switching off production of the sleep hormone melatonin. Our level of melatonin normally increases after darkness falls, making us feel drowsy. The SCN also governs functions that are synchronised with our sleep/wake cycle, including body temperature, hormone secretion, urine production and changes in blood pressure.

Our biological cycles normally follow the 24-hour cycle of the sun. For most of us a typical cycle means that we fall asleep at around 11pm and wake up seven to eight hours later between 6am and 8am. The more stable and consistent the cues given to our biological clock during the day and night, the better we will sleep. However, circadian rhythms can be affected to some degree by almost any kind of external time cue, such as the beeping of an alarm clock, the clatter of a rubbish truck, changes in temperature or the timing of meals.

WHAT WOULD HAPPEN IF YOU DIDN'T SLEEP?

Here's an overview of what research has shown can happen when your circadian rhythms are disrupted and you don't get the quality REM and non-REM sleep you need.

➤ **Bouts of drowsiness:** Inability to get through any day without an episode or episodes of energy loss or a dip in alertness, especially in the mid- to late afternoon. These bouts are most likely to occur after a meal, when sitting in a warm room or attending a boring lecture or meeting. Although these factors can trigger a dip in alertness they are not the cause of sleepiness during the day.

➤ **Loss of motivation:** Feelings of apathy or loss of motivation may occur, making it hard to complete tasks.

➤ **Reduced immunity:** The more sleep-deprived you are, the more likely you are to succumb to bouts of cold and flu as your immune system needs healthy sleep to function optimally.

➤ **Feeling shivery:** Feeling shivery or cold is often caused by trying to stay awake when your temperature plummets in preparation for sleep.

➤ **Weight gain:** Many sleep-deprived people consume foods high in sugar to help them stay awake, and this can lead to blood sugar imbalances and weight gain.

➤ **Reduced interaction:** Fatigue can make people reluctant to participate fully in group discussions or interactions with others.

➤ **Inability to cope:** Sleep-deprived people may find that they are often overwhelmed by feelings of helplessness when faced with tasks they could normally accomplish with ease. There may also be a loss of perspective and an inability to cope under pressure.

➤ **Mood swings:** Irritability and mood swings are common when people are tired; the threshold for anger lowers and this is one of the fastest ways to lose the respect of others.

➤ **Inattention:** Sleep-deprived people may fall asleep for brief moments and this can lead to accidents, misunderstandings and mistakes.

➤ **Reduced productivity:** Cognitive function and reaction time will be reduced. This can include reduced memory, concentration, creativity, coordination, decision making and communication skills, and an inability to think logically or critically or to assimilate new information.

If any of the above traits sound familiar, you are like the millions of other people who are not performing at their peak. Unfortunately, many of us are simply unaware that we are displaying some of these characteristics because we have got so used to bouts of drowsiness or low levels of energy that we think of it as normal. But normal it most certainly is not. We aren't meant to feel run down and tired during the day.

COMMON SYMPTOMS OF SLEEPLESS NIGHTS

➤ blurred vision
➤ irritability, edginess
➤ daytime drowsiness
➤ decreased mental activity and concentration
➤ weakened immune system
➤ dark circles under the eyes
➤ headaches
➤ loss of libido
➤ slow reaction time and memory loss
➤ nausea
➤ yawning

HOW MUCH SLEEP DO YOU NEED?

When pinned down, scientists say that between six and eight hours a night is enough for most of us. This is the basic amount of sleep we need to function comfortably in our daily life; beyond that, sleep is an enjoyable time-filler but is not essential. Just like sex and food, most of us would like to have more sleep than we need simply for enjoyment, not because it is good for our health.

Bear in mind that six to eight hours is the average amount of sleep a person needs. As pointed out in the previous chapter, your sleep needs will vary according to your individual circumstances. The key is to find out what works for you. If you feel alert and energetic during the day you are getting enough sleep for you; even if you are only sleeping five hours a night or as much as nine hours a night. If, however, you feel drowsy during the day and lacking in energy, the solution is simple: you need to improve the quality of your sleep.

Many of us try to make up for lost sleep by having long lie-ins on days off and weekends. In fact, these may be doing more harm than good, and I strongly advise against them. This isn't just because they disrupt your biological clock and make you prone to headaches, it's also because recent studies show that those who stay in bed for more than nine hours are more irritable and don't live as long as their eight-hour-sleep counterparts!

A 2002 study of more than a million people found that those who averaged eight or more hours of sleep a night had a 12 per cent greater chance of death than those who got six or seven. People who took sleeping pills were also more likely to die younger. Several studies since have reached the same conclusion but the reason is not clear.

DON'T KID YOURSELF

There's still so much to learn about the mystery of sleep but scientists are sending out clear messages to us that a good night's sleep is absolutely crucial if we want to look and feel good and think clearly. I think we'd be foolish to ignore these messages.

Perhaps you're a high-flier who thinks they don't need more than five hours a night? Don't kid yourself. You may be too drained to realise that you aren't performing at your peak. Whatever your age, profession or level of stamina, nobody can function properly without a good night's sleep. Contrary to popular opinion, you can't train yourself to need less sleep; you can only get used to it. This is as unproductive and damaging as getting used to feeling run down, tired and unhappy all the time.

WHAT HAPPENS IF YOU SLEEP FOR LESS THAN SIX HOURS?

A single all-nighter can vastly increase lapses of attention. Sleep researcher David Dinges at the University of Pennsylvania studied such lapses on pools of subjects who had slept for four, six or eight hours nightly for two weeks.

The researchers measured the subjects' speed of reaction to a computer screen where, at random intervals within a defined 10-minute period, the display would begin counting up in milliseconds from 000 to 1 second. The task was, first, to notice that the count had started and, second, to stop it as quickly as possible by hitting a key. It wasn't so much that the sleep-deprived subjects were slower, but that they had far more total lapses, letting the entire second go by without responding. Those on four hours a night had more lapses than those sleeping for six, who in turn had more lapses than subjects sleeping for eight hours per night.

In another study published in the British journal *Occupational and Environmental Medicine*, researchers in Australia and New Zealand reported that getting less than six hours' sleep a night can have some of the same hazardous effects as being drunk, affecting coordination, reaction time and judgement. Having less than six hours' sleep on a single night impairs motor skills such as reaction times, not to mention reverse parking. Staying awake for 17–19 hours affects your behind-the-wheel skills more than having a blood alcohol level of 0.05 per cent – the legal limit.

Without doubt, less than six hours' sleep impairs reaction time and performance on a wide variety of tasks. Many people argue that they get by just fine on very little sleep. However, research shows that only a tiny fraction of people can truly function well on less than seven hours' sleep per night. Moreover, people who chronically fail to get enough sleep may actually be cutting their lives short. A lack of sleep taxes the immune system, and may even lead to disease and premature ageing.

Sleep researcher Eve van Cauter at the University of Chicago exposed sleep-deprived students (allowed only four hours per night for six nights) to flu vaccine. Their immune systems produced only half the normal number of antibodies in response to the viral challenge. Levels of cortisol (a hormone associated with stress) rose, and the sympathetic nervous system became active, raising heart rates and blood pressure. The subjects also showed insulin resistance, a pre-diabetic condition that affects glucose tolerance and produces weight gain. According to van Cauter, when 18-year-olds are restricted to four hours' sleep a night, within a couple of weeks their ability to metabolise glucose is similar to that of a 60-year-old.

To make all of this worse, most people who are sleep-deprived do not even realise it. This is because when you live on less than six hours a night you forget what it's like to be really awake.

Perhaps you do want to get a good night's sleep but simply can't. Many of my clients would love nothing better than eight hours of uninterrupted sleep but just can't make it through the night for a variety of reasons, so I try to help them ensure that the sleep they do get is good quality. The next chapter will take a look at why sleep has become an impossible dream for so many people these days and what factors are keeping us awake at night.

THREE

Why Can't I Get a Good Night's Sleep?

As a physiotherapist, it is clear to me that back problems, snoring partners and beds long past their sell by date are common causes of poor quality sleep. However, none of these problems is the reason why sleep deprivation has become a modern epidemic. The real reason is the 24/7 world we now live in.

It seems that the invention of the electric light bulb was a double-edged sword: earlier light sources weren't strong enough to permit people to read or work comfortably late into the night. Ever since the first bulb shed its light we have been detaching ourselves from our natural rhythms. Now, ever-increasing business hours and longer journeys to work cut into our precious free time. We face endless distractions to keep us out of bed in the evenings, and the simple truth is that our biological clocks can't always keep up with seemingly endless days and non-existent nights.

Today's 24-hour economy pushes hardworking people to work longer hours without giving them proper information on the effects of sleep deprivation, and how it can lead to accidents, injury and depression.

'I'm an investment banker and I used to think being short on sleep was part of my job. I make sleep a priority now but I can remember going a whole day and night without sleep and, can you believe it, actually starting to nod off during a meeting with my boss to review my performance.'
MARK, 35

SLEEP DEBT

Some people think that a sleep debt is like an overdrawn bank account, and that a built-up debt can be repaid simply by catching up on sleep at weekends or days off. This popular understanding of sleep debt and how to pay it off is not wholly accurate. For instance, if you typically sleep for eight hours a night and only get six you can recover the two-hour debt the following night. However, if you keep missing two hours of sleep a night your sleep debt becomes chronic, and chronic sleep debt can lead to poor health. Trying to catch up on sleep on odd days off isn't going to help if you're chronically sleep deprived; in fact, it could make things worse by disrupting your circadian rhythms (*see Chapter 2, page 12*). Your best option is to skip the lie-in, go to bed earlier and wake up at the same time every day, including weekends and days off.

DIY SLEEP ASSESSMENT

If catching up on sleep during holidays and weekends isn't the answer, how can you cancel your sleep debt? The following three quizzes will help you assess how sleep-deprived you are, what may be stopping you getting the quality sleep you need, and whether or not you have a sleep disorder.

QUIZ: ARE YOU SLEEP-DEPRIVED?

Which, if any, of the following apply to you?

1. You need an alarm clock to wake you up.
2. You fall asleep within five minutes of getting into bed.
3. You sleep longer and better at the weekends.
4. You have trouble getting out of bed in the mornings.
5. You experience drowsiness during the day, especially around 4pm.
6. You doze off while watching television.
7. You doze off after a heavy lunch.
8. You yawn excessively.
9. You need caffeine and stimulants to get through the day.
10. You doze off in public places such as a meeting at work.
11. You doze off while driving.
12. You suffer from early-morning headaches.
13. You have dark circles or bags under the eyes.
14. You have trouble concentrating.
15. You have problems remembering things.

If three or more items on the list from 1 to 8 apply to you and/or one or more items from 9 to 15, this suggests a lack of good quality sleep. You are not alone, but even though fatigue is commonplace, don't make the mistake of thinking that tiredness is something you simply have to learn to live with. Yes, it is possible to train yourself to get by on less sleep but during sleep your body and brain are restored, rejuvenated and re-energised, so why would you skimp on such a valuable resource?

Many working professionals assume that they are good sleepers because they fall asleep the minute their head hits the pillow but this is a clear sign of sleep deprivation. The well-rested person takes 15–20 minutes to fall asleep. So if you are getting less than six to eight hours' sleep a night, or if you need an alarm clock to wake up, or if you fall asleep the moment your head touches the pillow, you are sleep-deprived and unaware of how alert and energetic you would feel with enough sleep.

Another common misconception is that feeling sleepy during boring meetings or in a warm room or after a heavy lunch is perfectly normal but not one of these situations causes sleepiness. In fact, if you've had enough sleep things like dull meetings can still make you feel bored but not sleepy.

Catching up

Don't get anxious if you are a little sleep-deprived now and again, but if you often feel sluggish and drowsy during the day you are not performing to your potential and need to establish a healthy sleep routine. Here's what you need to do:

➤ On working days establish a regular sleeping and waking time that allows a minimum of six to eight hours of sleep a night.

➤ If you feel the need to catch up on sleep at weekends and on days off, go to bed earlier than usual and sleep until you wake up naturally. Don't lie in bed once you have woken up.

➤ Read the advice in Chapters 4 to 7 to make absolutely sure you are doing all you can to ensure you get a good night's sleep.

➤ Review the advice in Chapters 9, 10 and 11 to see if any physical problems are interfering with the quality of your sleep, and Chapter 12 to see if your diet is the culprit.

➤ Pay specific attention to Chapter 8: The Power of Napping.

QUIZ: HOW HEALTHY IS YOUR SLEEP STRATEGY?

Answer yes or no to the following:

1. Do you go to bed and wake up at different times depending on your schedule?
2. Do you enjoy long lie-ins at the weekend?
3. Do you have caffeinated drinks or alcohol after 4pm?
4. Has it been a few years since you bought a new bed or mattress?
5. When you can't fall asleep do you just lie there and try harder?
6. Do you watch television or surf the net before you go to bed?
7. Does your partner's tossing and turning or snoring keep you awake?
8. Do you take over-the-counter medication to help you fall asleep?
9. Is your bedroom too warm and/or noisy?
10. Do you sleep on your back or stomach?
11. Do you wake up with back or neck ache?

If you answered yes to three or more of the questions above, certain aspects of your lifestyle are making it impossible for you to get a good night's sleep. Fortunately, there are many things you can do to make sure your sleep strategies and your sleep are sound. The following guidelines will help:

➤ Avoid long lie-ins and establish a regular sleeping and waking time that allows you at least six to eight hours of sleep a night, and stick to that pattern. In other words, get up at the same time and try to go to bed at the same time each day. Remember, sleeping in for long periods at holidays and weekends is not the answer because this means your normal waking time will be shifted, making it harder for you to sleep the next night. If you do feel the need to sleep longer to catch up for a series of late nights, try to do so by going to bed earlier than usual for three to four weeks, even if you like to burn the midnight oil.

➤ Work through Chapters 4 to 7 to see if the advice will solve your sleep problems. Many people find that their problems are easily solved by a change in their bedroom environment.

➤ Review the advice in Chapter 12 to ensure that your diet is optimum for good sleep, and see Chapters 9, 10 and 11 to check whether physical problems are interfering with the quality of your sleep.

➤ If your partner is making it hard for you to get a good night's sleep, see Chapter 14.

QUIZ: DO YOU HAVE A SLEEP DISORDER?

Answer yes or no to the following:

1. Do you wake up a number of times in the night?
2. Do you have trouble falling asleep most nights?
3. When you wake up in the night, is it hard to fall back to sleep?
4. Have you been told that you snore very loudly?
5. Do you find it extremely difficult to wake up in the morning?
6. Do you get a tingling sensation in your legs when you go to sleep?
7. Do you sleepwalk or move excessively in your sleep?
8. Do you sometimes wake up anxious and scared in the night and don't know why?

If you answered yes to any of these questions, Chapters 9 and 10 offer practical solutions to common problems that can interfere with sleep. If none of this helps, you may have a sleep disorder and should refer to the advice in Chapter 11. (*For sleeping problems associated with jet lag and shift work, see Chapter 15.*)

NIGHT OWLS AND LARKS

Larks are morning types who like to get up early and go to bed early. They perform at their best before midday. Owls, on the other hand, don't have high energy levels in the morning and come alive in the evening. Sleep characteristics are genetically determined, which makes it difficult to change your natural sleeping pattern. You can work around them, however, depending on your job and lifestyle (*see box, below*).

Age-old beliefs that larks are somehow healthier or superior in some way to owls are incorrect. Although there are indications that early to bed, early to rise can be more beneficial, research has also shown that as long as the sleep you get is restorative it doesn't matter when you sleep.

ADVICE FOR OWLS

➤ Use an alarm clock to help you get up in the morning.
➤ Drink a glass of energy-boosting lemon juice or fruit juice on waking.
➤ Soon after waking expose yourself to bright light to reset your biological clock.

➤ Make sure you always eat breakfast; eggs on wholemeal toast are a wonderful way to start the day, or try a bowl of oatmeal porridge sprinkled with nuts and seeds.

➤ If you can, exercise in your lunch hour or in the early afternoon.

➤ Try not to nap during the day.

➤ Eat a lighter evening meal.

➤ Don't always be the last to leave the party.

➤ Surf the internet and watch television earlier in the evening.

ADVICE FOR LARKS

➤ If your energy dips mid-afternoon try taking a 20-minute nap.

➤ Exercise in the early evening but not within two hours of bedtime.

➤ Get plenty of fresh air and daylight during the afternoon if you need to stay up late.

➤ Avoid alcohol in the evening.

➤ Have a healthy dessert if you find yourself flagging when you are out at dinner.

KEY POINTS

➤ We need between six and eight hours of sleep a night; no more, no less. Less than six hours triples our risk of a car accident but more than nine hours is associated with an increased risk of depression and poor health.

➤ If you can, try to go to bed before 11pm when physiological repair work is at its height.
➤ Get up at the same time each day or soon after you wake up naturally. Long lie-ins at the weekend when you fall asleep again after waking up naturally upset your biological clock and make things worse.
➤ The odd sleepless night or restless period is not a disaster, it's perfectly normal. It's also fine to enjoy the odd lie-in.
➤ Make quality sleep a priority, however hectic your lifestyle.

FOUR

Bed MOT

The bed that's right for you may be entirely different to the bed that's right for someone else. It really is important to be aware of the best bed, mattress and pillow for you and your build. For instance, if you are nine stone and petite, your bed needs will be very different to those of a 14-stone, muscular person.

If you find yourself waking up with aches and pains or stiffness that goes by mid-morning of its own accord, your bed is almost certainly causing you problems and you won't be getting a quality night's sleep. Another clear sign that you need a bed MOT is when you realise you slept better somewhere other than home. For example, you've just come back from holiday or a business conference and noticed how comfortable the hotel bed was. Hotels use the quality of their beds and bedding as marketing tools in their advertising. Although they're not usually top of the range, hotel mattresses do get changed almost every other year.

TIME FOR A NEW BED?

Buying a new bed may give you a better night's sleep than taking a sleeping pill! Two-year research by sleep expert Dr Chris Idzikowski found that those with uncomfortable beds slept on average one hour less each night than those with comfortable beds.

The question I'm probably asked most by my clients with sleeping problems is: should I buy a new bed? To find out if it is time for you to purchase a new bed, answer the following questions:

➤ Is your bed eight years old or more?
➤ Do you ever wake up with an aching neck or back?
➤ When lying in bed, do you feel springs, hardness or ridges beneath the surface?
➤ When moving in bed do you hear creaks, crunches or other strange noises?
➤ Do you and your partner roll towards each other unintentionally?
➤ Do your legs or arms dangle over the side of the bed when you sleep?
➤ Is the mattress or base uneven or sagging?
➤ Are the legs and castors worn out?
➤ Would it be embarrassing if your friends saw the bed without its covers?
➤ Is the mattress cover torn or stained?
➤ Does your mattress feel lumpy, soft, too hard or uncomfortable?
➤ Does your mattress sag in the middle or at the sides?
➤ Are there sagging spots around the edges or where you usually lie?

If your answer to two or more of the above questions is 'yes' it's definitely time to make a great investment for your future and buy a new bed, or to make changes to your current bed.

Ideally, you should renew your bed and mattress every five to eight years. If your bed is over eight years old you will almost certainly need to buy a new bed and mattress. If, however, your bed is under eight years old the advice below will help you fix your current bed.

HOW TO FIX YOUR EXISTING BED

Advice on buying a new bed is provided below. However, if buying a new bed is not an option for you, and you have to make do with your existing bed, there are certain things you can do to ease the strain and improve your chances of a good night's sleep.

If your bed feels too soft you need to find ways to make it firmer. Putting some plywood underneath your mattress can make a real difference. This is available from DIY stores, and you'll need a piece approximately 2 x 1 metres (6 x 3 feet). Alternatively, any firm surface can be used to harden the bed. If these measures don't work you always have the option of putting the mattress on the floor, but make sure you get help lifting it, especially if you suffer from back problems.

If your partner is a lot heavier or lighter than you, the answer is to put two single mattresses of different density on one base. This will, for example, stop your partner rolling into you if they are 16 stone and you are 9 stone. Alternatively, you can hook two separate beds together.

If your bed feels too hard, get an extra duvet, fold it in half and lie on top of it. Pillows placed under the arch of your back and your knees will help too. You can also buy mattress softeners (or toppers as they are sometimes called) from bed shops or ask for some foam to be cut to size. Do make sure you put the mattress softener/topper on top of your mattress and not under it.

MATTRESS TOPPERS

Mattress manufacturers are well aware that not everyone can afford to buy a mattress every five to eight years. A mattress topper is an affordable solution. It provides a comfortable, supportive layer that sits on top of your mattress underneath your bottom sheet and protects your mattress at the same time. It can be used with other bed accessories or your mattress provided you've carefully checked the manufacturer's instructions for both items. You can buy mattress toppers at any bed retailer, and they come in all sizes and depths. They may be made of memory foam or filled with polyester or natural fillings, such as duck feather and down. Mattress enhancers are normally thicker than mattress protectors and may be an inch or more thick (25 mm).

If you have a very firm bed and mattress and you're finding they don't give you the level of comfort you're looking for, a thick mattress topper may help. The additional layer, sometimes made from memory foam (visco-elastic) or similar material, will reduce the firmness and mould to your body, giving you the additional support you need.

Foam mattress toppers made from a unique kind of foam come from NASA research into materials that provide the right support for astronauts. The heat from your body helps the foam adapt to your sleeping position, supporting you exactly where you need it. When you get up and the foam stops sensing your body temperature, it reverts to its natural state. When you move during the night, the foam adjusts with you, providing you with the same support, no matter what position you're sleeping in.

A NEW BED OR A NEW MATTRESS?

If you already have a wood or metal bedstead in good condition you may only need a new mattress as bedsteads tend to be more hardwearing. If you have a divan, however, a new mattress alone won't give you the full benefit, and I strongly advise you to replace both.

If your bed is over eight years old – whether you have a bedstead or a divan – the base will be getting tired. There is a saying within the bed trade that a 'base will outlive one mattress but not two'. The best advice is always to try and buy base and mattress together because the two are designed and manufactured to complement one another in terms of support. Your mattress may be showing visible signs of wear and tear but the base will have had equal pressure and strain – it just doesn't show quite so clearly. Also, if you purchase from different manufacturers any warranty may be compromised if the manufacturer deems the base to be unsuitable to support the mattress, or vice versa. Another point to watch is making sure the dimensions of any separately sourced base and mattress are compatible – two kings might not be quite the same size.

A new bed and mattress set may not be a wonder cure for all life's stresses and strains, but it certainly should help you get a better night's sleep, leaving you refreshed and ready to face the world. And don't let the hassle of getting rid of your old bed put you off buying a new one; many bed retailers take away your old bed for a small fee, and one leading bed retailer has recently announced that it is investing one million pounds in bed recycling machines so you can dispose of your old bed in an eco-friendly way for a small charge.

BUYING A NEW BED

'I never realised how important buying a good bed was until I got a bad back!' MARTIN, 27

What's the difference between memory foam and latex? Are latex mattresses too hot? What price should I pay for a good bed? How do I tell if a mattress is going to be comfortable? What bed should I buy?

These are just some of the questions clients ask me when they start shopping for beds. There are literally thousands of beds from which to choose, and I always tell my clients to ignore any advertising hype and choose a bed that meets their needs. There's no such thing as the perfect bed for a particular condition or situation, such as an ideal bed for a back pain sufferer. Although a good retailer will arm you with lots of information to make the process simpler, only you can make the final, important decision – so take your time and make it wisely, choosing a bed that meets your needs. If you suffer from backache or other aches and pains, consult a physiotherapist before making your purchase.

As buying a new bed is one of the most important decisions you can make for your health and wellbeing, it's important to know what you are looking for before you part with your money. The information below will help.

BUYING A NEW BED: SEVEN EASY STEPS

1: Set Your Budget

As with most things, the price of a bed set does not necessarily tell you how comfortable it will be. Beds are priced from several hundreds of pounds to thousands, but the most expensive is not necessarily the best for you as comfort is a matter of individual preference. A very firm, expensive bed may be uncomfortable if you prefer a softer mattress, for example. Bear in mind, however, that more expensive beds will use better quality materials and fillings. If you think about the cost of a bed over its lifetime – say approximately 10 years – then the cost per night is minimal. A £750 bed would only be about 20 pence a night over 10 years – not much when you think about it! The best thing you can do is buy the best bed you can afford. Your bed is an investment, and how well you sleep affects the quality of your life. Don't skimp, but set your budget and stick to it.

2: Size Matters

I recommend buying a bed about 15 cm (6 inches) longer than you are, if possible. A single bed should not be less than 90 cm (35 inches) wide and a double bed not less than 160 cm (63 inches). We turn about 20–40 times a night and need the room to move freely. The size of your room is one factor to consider and you need room to walk around your bed so that you can get in and out of it easily.

Another thing to think about is whether you'll be sleeping alone. If so, any size bed will work as long as it is 15 cm (6 inches) longer than you; but if you are sharing the bed you should choose the biggest bed possible. Most standard double beds give both partners less room than a single bed each would. Bear in mind, too, that bed sizes are not standard, and a king size in one shop may be different from a king size in another. The table below lists standard bed sizes but this is no guarantee that the standard applies in every retailer, so do check first.

COMMON NAME	USUAL SIZE (METRIC)	USUAL SIZE (IMPERIAL)
Single	90 x 190 cm	3 ft x 6 ft 3 in
Double	135 x 190 cm	4 ft 6 in x 6 ft 3 in
King	150 x 200 cm	5 ft x 6 ft 6 in
Super King	180 x 200 cm	6 ft x 6 ft 6 in

3: Decide Type and Style

Bedsteads are usually made from wood or metal and there are many variations and colours to choose from. They are more decorative and will provide a definite classic or contemporary look to your bedroom. A 'bowed slat' (or 'sprung slat') bedstead will give more cushioned support than 'solid slat', which has a firmer feel.

Divans act as bases for mattresses and either have springs which allow the mattress to adapt to the body's contours, or a solid top which provides firmer support. A divan is useful if you're tight on space as most are available with drawers to provide additional storage. Bear in mind that a divan may have drawers or storage which involve lifting a heavy bed and may therefore not be suitable for anyone with low back pain.

Futons are mattresses, usually without springs, that are supported by a wooden or metal frame that can fold into a sofa during the day and open as a bed at night. The mattresses must be very flexible, so they are typically made of cotton, synthetic fibres and foam in various combinations. The futon is designed to support sitting as well as sleeping but I recommend them only for occasional use as all the lifting and bending to make and unmake the bed can cause lower back strain and distort the mattress.

Electrically adjustable beds allow sleepers to adjust the head and foot of the bed to the most comfortable position. The mattress and foundation must be specially built for the flexing motion and can be innerspring, foam or a combination. Since the flexing causes extra wear on the mattress, quality construction is very important. Mattresses not built for this purpose should not be used with an adjustable bed frame. You also need to bear in mind that however much a bed adjusts, this is no guarantee that it will meet your needs or optimise your sleeping posture. Finally, your posture will be affected if you are using the electrics to put you in a slumped posture, and it is not ideal to fall asleep upright unless you have a particular medical condition.

Most **waterbeds** are now designed to look like normal divans, with a water-filled core providing support coupled with layers of upholstery for insulation and surface comfort. Quality construction is especially critical when water is involved, so look for assurance that the vinyl and seaming are designed for maximum durability.

Although you can get specially-made **orthopaedic mattresses**, many manufacturers provide firmer, supportive mattresses that give the spine the protection and pressure reduction it needs. These mattresses are often manufactured with a high coil count, making them slightly firmer and more responsive to the position and movement of the sleeper. Although orthopaedic beds work for some people, I want to stress that they are not always beneficial, and can sometimes make problems worse. So if you don't want to end up with an empty pocket and back pain, research your options carefully.

Airbeds are now designed to look like the familiar mattress/bedstead combination, with an air-filled core providing the support instead of an innerspring unit or foam core. These designs also offer a range of feels and typically are adjustable to suit individual sleeper's needs. Bear in mind, however, that airbeds are suitable only for temporary use.

Headboards are optional and purely decorative. Most divans are sold without them so you have a choice.

4: Go for a Test Drive

You wouldn't buy a car without a test drive; so don't buy a bed without lying in it first or getting your partner, if you have one, to lie in it with you. You should always visit a shop to try out a bed before ordering. Never order your bed online or by phone unless you have tried it out in the store first.

It's no good simply pushing your hands on the mattress or sitting down on the bed; you need to see what it feels like to lie down on it. Slip off your shoes, take off your coat or jacket and ask the salesperson to give you some time to lie down in your normal sleeping position. When you are lying down look for a mattress and foundation set that supports your body at all points. If you aren't getting enough support you'll get back pain, and a mattress that is too hard can create uncomfortable pressure after lying in the same position for around 10 minutes. So make sure you lie down for five minutes at least on a bed to see if it is supporting you properly before moving on to the next one.

When you lie down, slide your hands gently under your lower back. If there is a lot of space the mattress is too hard, and if there is no space it is too soft. What you need is just enough space to slide your hand comfortably but snugly in between your back and the mattress.

5: Buy a Mattress that Moulds to Your Body

Another question I'm often asked is, 'Should I get a soft or a hard mattress?' In fact, thinking that they want a firm mattress is the number one mistake people make. Super-firm mattresses are actually a detriment to most people. What you want is a mattress that moulds to your body and supports you so there is no undue pressure anywhere. Each one of us has different needs and wants.

There is nothing wrong with a soft mattress as long as it gives you adequate support, especially in the small of your back when you lie on your back. A mattress that is too hard can't do this. The ideal mattress should keep your spine in alignment and distribute pressure evenly throughout your body, making uninterrupted contact with it. A mattress has to be soft enough to fill in the gap under your lower back but not so soft that it sags completely under your weight.

When it comes to spring type the greater the number or thickness of the springs, the firmer the mattress. Mattress firmness is rated from one to five, with five being the firmest. A rating between three and four is generally best for most of us, but again you need to find what works best for you. Women, especially those with hour-glass figures, tend to need softer mattresses, and men with fewer contours to their body prefer firmer mattresses. How much you weigh should also be taken into consideration.

The amount of padding on the mattress determines the level of comfort. Adding a mattress topper to a firm mattress may be a good choice for some individuals with back pain.

6: Check What's Inside Your Mattress

What is inside your mattress matters a lot so you need to ask a salesperson about the construction process and fillings used. There are many different kinds of filling, and a combination of some or all can radically alter the feel of each mattress. They can also radically alter the price.

Sprung mattresses are constructed around a series of coils or springs. They are designed to provide the support the sleeper needs without any discomfort, and are built to last as long as possible. Different manufacturers design and make their sprung mattresses in different ways, but the principle is the same. Open spring is the most popular spring type. Continuous spring is where the springs are made from a single piece of wire, giving a more responsive feel. The springs also run from head to toe, rather than from side to side, stopping you from rolling over while you're asleep. Pocket sprung mattresses have small springs that are sewn into individual pockets, making the mattress more responsive to the weight and position of the sleeper. The more springs there are, the more individual support the mattress can give.

Non-sprung mattresses don't simply contain springs. Their construction can be from a wide variety of materials, and research and technology are constantly refining the ways that manufacturers can provide consumers with the very best mattresses. Popular construction materials include latex, fibre, wool, cotton, foam and even water.

Latex beds are made from the natural sap of rubber trees and are often considered a luxury, although they are good for allergy sufferers as dust mites cannot survive within them. However, women with hormonal problems, or going through the menopause, may find that a latex bed makes hot flushes feel worse as they can get very warm. This is because a latex mattress conforms so well to your body contours that it may provide a greater degree of insulation than any other mattress.

Coir fibre is a popular filling material, usually packed around the springs to keep them in place. Coir fibre is 100 per cent natural and is made from coconut husks. It is used for many other purposes, but is a mainstay filling for the mattress industry.

Wool is used for its luxury feel, but it also has natural properties that make it an excellent mattress filling. Naturally breathable, it is also resilient and has fire-retardant properties.

Cotton, silk and cashmere are at the luxury end of the market. These materials are soft, fine and natural, making for the perfect finish to a top-of-the-range product.

Foam is used as a filling in some mattresses and as the core of the mattress in others. There are various types of foam in use. Some manufacturers use foam that recoils and reacts to the temperature of your body to create a moulded, supportive mattress; for example, memory foam is very popular (one of my clients said 'It's like sleeping on a cloud.') but its temperature and resistance can vary (it can become hard in cold temperatures, and some menopausal women find it a little too hot).

Other foams are used in conjunction with springs to provide the ultimate in mattress comfort. Although current mattress technology means that sprung mattresses and other fillings are more supportive than ever, they may not always provide the level of support you're looking for. Foam might not suit everyone, and isn't a miracle bed, but this kind of mattress may give you the 'weightless' feeling you're looking for if you have a bad back, or regularly wake up with aches and pains.

7: Check What's on the Outside

The mattress cover is one of the most important parts. It's built to hold the mattress together, to protect it from general wear and tear and to make you feel as comfortable as possible. For this reason, the cover (ticking) tends to be made from tough cotton or viscose yarns, and the material is often treated against stains and allergens. Look out for the following:

➤ **Pillow top:** an extra layer on the mattress top that gives a super-soft finish.
➤ **Hand-tufted:** a traditional way of finishing the mattress that 'buttons' the filling to the mattress cover for a firmer finish.
➤ **Micro quilt:** secures the filling to the cover in a raised quilted pattern, creating a softer feel.
➤ **Latex:** a layer of breathable natural rubber is placed on top of the springs to protect against dust mites, and to mould to your body shape for extra comfort.

MAKING YOUR DECISION

Natalie, 32, moved into unfurnished rented accommodation six years ago and rushed out to buy a flat-pack bed which she assembled herself. It was a bargain price with next day delivery, and Natalie didn't have the time to wait *for a bed to be delivered in four to six weeks. For the past six months Natalie has been waking at night feeling uncomfortable, and most mornings she wakes up with a stiff, sore lower back. It takes her a while to get going. At first she thought exercising in the morning was causing the problem but when she discussed it with me it became apparent that it was her lumpy, soft, unsupportive bed that was the source of the strain. I advised her to put her current mattress on the floor and order a firm-to-medium bed. Natalie's new bed arrived four weeks later and within two weeks of its arrival Natalie noticed a reduction in her night time discomfort, morning stiffness and soreness, and even felt confident to restart her morning exercise.*

The type of mattress you eventually choose will depend on the style you find most comfortable. That's why you should try both sprung and non-sprung mattresses of various types before you buy. A recoil foam mattress may not sound appealing to you, but you may change your mind once you've tried it and felt how it moulds to your shape and provides the ideal support. The same applies to the latest pocket sprung mattresses and any other styles that you try.

On the outside look for fine tailoring, superior fabrics and a surface that looks quality-made. Lift up the mattress and have a good look at the base because this is where the first economies are made. Then give the bed a good shake. If it feels rickety in the shop, what will it be like in a couple of years' time?

HOW TO CARE FOR YOUR MATTRESS

After delivery your mattress should be aired for four hours to freshen it and remove any aroma from storage. The mattress should also be aired on a weekly basis by turning back the bed linen for a few hours.

With sprung mattresses it's important to turn your mattress every two weeks to maximise its life. Body weight compresses a mattress, leading to dips and ultimately an uneven sleeping surface. Consider a one-sided 'no-turn' mattress if turning a heavy mattress could be difficult. Latex and recoil foam mattresses do not need turning, and in some cases have only one sleeping surface so cannot be turned, but the mattress should still be rotated lengthways occasionally (once a month) to maximise its life. Over time, these mattresses may feel as if they are gradually getting softer, as cells within the foam open more fully and the surface reacts more quickly. However, the important pressure-relieving properties remain the same, and eventually the whole mattress will react evenly.

Use a mattress protector or an under-blanket below the sheet. (Avoid using a plastic sheet on or under the mattress as this prevents air circulation and can cause condensation.) A mattress protector helps prolong the life of the mattress, protects it from staining and alleviates dust and mite infestation. Your body loses over a quarter of a litre of moisture per night and half a kilo of dead skin a year. It is therefore very unhygienic not to have a protective, washable barrier like a mattress protector. You also increase the risk of having an allergic reaction to the build-up of dust mites.

Don't sit on the edge of your mattress. Mattresses are designed to spread the weight over a wide area. It's also not a good idea to walk or jump on your bed or to bend or roll it as this could all cause serious damage to the spring unit and tear the material.

DUST MITES

Your mattress is one of the key places that dust mites like to live. It's warm, cosy and constantly fed with the fluid and dead skin that we lose at night. In many cases, it's the enzymes released in dust mite droppings that cause or inflame allergic reactions – particularly asthma or other breathing problems. There are things you can do to keep your mattress as free from dust mites as possible.

Humidity: Dust mites love high humidity. Mites are rare in dry climates unless the use of evaporative coolers adds moisture to the air. Reduce humidity in your home by ventilating your house often, and try to get rid of steam after bathing or while cooking by opening the windows and letting plenty of dry air into the house.

Hygiene: It's important that you keep your bed and your bedroom as hygienic as you can. Don't make your bed in the morning – let it air for at least 20 minutes, preferably for the whole day. Dust mites dislike cold air and light, so leaving your bed unmade produces the conditions they hate. Wash your bedding once a week and use a hot wash every so often as this helps kill off any dust mites that may be in your bedding.

Covers: Buying mattress and pillow covers won't remove dust mites completely, but it will reduce the conditions for breeding and also help to prevent so much allergen being released into the air. As part of a dust mite reduction programme, you should have mattress and pillow covers for all the beds in your home. When you change the bed, leave the mattress exposed for at least half an hour to air.

Cleaning: Whilst vacuuming your mattress won't remove the dust mites, it will remove some of the dust they feed on. Make sure you vacuum carefully so that you don't damage the mattress itself. Carpets and curtains also harbour dust mites, so you may want to consider installing wooden or other flooring and blinds instead of curtains. Clean your room regularly and air it, even in winter.

Mattress doctor: Check at your local bed store to see if there is a mattress cleaner in your area who can come and give your mattress a good clean and vacuum every six months.

BEDDING IN

I often tell my clients not to instantly expect the perfect night's sleep after buying a new bed. Just like a new pair of shoes or jeans, your new bed will take some time to get used to so don't expect to have the night of your dreams immediately. You need to give the fillings in your new mattress time to settle and compress, and it typically takes three to four weeks before you will get used to and feel truly comfortable in your brand-new bed.

BED-BUYING DO'S AND DON'TS

➤ **Do** lie down on the bed; both of you if it's two of you.

➤ **Do** take off your shoes and coat and lie in your normal sleeping position.

➤ **Do** ask for advice and information on each bed.

➤ **Do** buy a mattress that moulds to your body.

➤ **Don't** just prod the mattress with your fingers.

➤ **Don't** be embarrassed to lie on the bed.

➤ **Don't** buy on price alone.

➤ **Don't** buy in a hurry – remember, this is a long-term investment you are making for your future health and wellbeing.

FIVE

Pillows and Bedclothes

PILLOW TALK

In my experience as a physiotherapist, not only do I trial most pillows on the market but I also ask my clients to bring their pillows into my practice so that I can assess the condition of their pillows and whether they need to be replaced and whether they are being used correctly.

A good pillow is just as important as a good bed for getting a good night's sleep. Even though we rarely give a lot of thought to the pillows we use, buying the right pillow and positioning it correctly could be one of the most important parts of sleeping success. It is a very comforting feeling to have just the right pillow to rest an achy, tired body on. In addition to providing comfort, the right pillows can also give the necessary support for the neck and spine, alleviating or preventing many common forms of back and neck pain.

PILLOW MOT

I have seen many back and neck problems aggravated, if not caused, by bad or worn-out pillows. If your pillow is six months old or more it could need replacing. Assuming normal use and wear and tear, a polyester pillow lasts for six months to two years, a down pillow five years and a feather pillow eight years. If, however, your pillow is clearly showing signs of wear, such as loss of shape and flatness, it is time to shop for a new pillow.

If you aren't sure if it's time to replace your pillow, test the support of down and feather pillows by laying the fluffed pillow on a hard surface. Fold it in half or thirds and squeeze out the air. Release the pillow. If it unfolds and returns to its original position, it has support; a broken pillow will stay folded. To test the support of a polyester pillow, fluff and fold as above. Then place a weight of around 300g (10 ounces), such as a trainer, on the pillow. A pillow with support will unfold itself and throw off the shoe; a broken pillow will stay folded.

BUYING A NEW PILLOW

For a better night's sleep the pillow that is best for you is one that you can squish and fluff to meet your contours and sleeping position. Your pillow should fit you like a glove. Your goal when buying a new pillow is to know what pillow firmness is going to allow your neck and spine to be aligned properly so there is no gap between your neck and the mattress.

The traditional pillow is the mattress top pillow, used to provide support for the head, neck and upper spine while the body is lying in bed in a resting position. When determining the number of pillows to use, bear in mind that too many tilt your head forwards and too few tilt your head backwards if you lie on your back. Similarly, if lying on your side, be sure the gap between your head and shoulders is filled by pillow. Find a balance that enables you to maintain the midline position. For optimum support, it is best to select a pillow that has the following characteristics:

Designed to Keep the Spine in Natural Alignment
The human neck curves slightly forwards (to sustain the weight of the head when upright), and it's important to maintain this curve when in a lying position. If the pillow is too high when

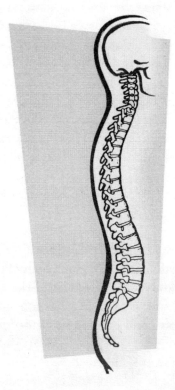

sleeping on your side or on your back, the neck is bent abnormally forwards or to the side, causing muscle strain on the back of the neck and shoulders. This type of position may also cause narrowing of the air pipe, resulting in obstructed breathing, and sometimes snoring, which can hinder sleep. Conversely, if the height of the pillow is too low, the neck muscles can also be strained.

The amount and type of support you need from your pillow (whether it be one, one and a half or two pillows) depends on your sleeping position as well as your weight and the density of your mattress, but always try to consider the depth of your shoulder in comparison to the distance from your head to the bed. You need to fill that large area with a pillow, thus providing an equal surface to position your head so that it is even with your spine. In short, the pillow should maintain an approximate height of 10–15 cm (4–6 inches), properly supporting the head and neck.

For correct sleeping posture, only your head and neck should be placed over your pillow. Do not place your shoulders on the pillow because this will elevate your upper body much higher than your lower body. You could try rolling up a hand towel and placing it in your pillow to fill the gap between your neck and shoulder. To maintain the balance of the entire body, the sleeper can place a pillow between bent knees to achieve the midline position when lying on their side.

Comfortable

A large part of what makes a good pillow is personal preference. If the pillow feels comfortable, it's likely to help you relax, get a good night's sleep and feel well-rested in the morning. The pillow's surface can also be a source of comfort – some people prefer a pillowcase with a cool, smooth feeling (such as cotton), while others prefer warmth (such as flannel). The pillow filling is also a matter of personal preference.

Adjustable

To help the pillow conform to various sleep positions, it is best if the pillow can be adjusted to fit the unique shape, curves and sleeping position of the user. A pillow should mould to one's individual shape and alleviate any pressure points.

PILLOWS FOR DIFFERENT SLEEPING POSITIONS

When shopping for a new pillow, buy at least two pillows as they can be used to support other parts of your body as well as the head and neck.

Sleeping on your back: Your pillow should support the natural curvature of your spine; there should also be adequate support under your head, neck and shoulders. Placing a pillow or two beneath the knees further alleviates any back strain, and is the gentlest position for the back. This position can help you drift off to sleep but bear in mind that during the night the pillows may move as you move, and if you wake up you will need to reposition them.

Sleeping on your side: When lying on your side, the pillow should support your head and neck so that your spine maintains the midline position. Weight should be evenly distributed so as not to create unnatural bending or pressure. Some people may like to place a small pillow or rolled-up towel under their waist for additional support while lying on their side, especially if they have an hourglass figure.

Sleeping on your stomach: When sleeping or resting on your stomach, your pillow should be relatively flat or removed. This will help keep your spine in line and enable you to sleep better. In this position, it is often best to place another relatively flat pillow under your stomach to help the spine keep its natural alignment. If your mattress is soft you may well need to place more than one pillow under your stomach. They will help minimise the amount of strain on your lower back as well as the amount of twisting for your neck.

PILLOW TYPES

Filling

The fill of the pillow you choose is important. Different fills provide different advantages and degrees of firmness, and they can range in price from tens to hundreds of pounds. Again, the right pillow for you depends on your budget and your individual needs.

Naturally filled pillows, such as down or feather pillows, give you comfort and adjustability. They can support your head, eliminate pressure points and increase facial circulation to decrease face squashing. Down pillows are the ultimate in comfort and luxury. However, if your pillow has any chance of becoming damp – such as in an extremely humid area or in a camper van or boat – it may not be the best option as it can develop an odour. Down is also not an option if you suffer from asthma or have allergies.

Cotton-filled pillows are available in a range of thicknesses and comfort levels. If you can pinpoint the proper combination you require, a cotton-filled pillow is an ideal choice. They also have the benefit of working well for people with allergies.

Foam-filled pillows are inexpensive. They are often of lower quality than your average pillow with a less comforting, luxurious feel. They come in a range of fills from solid to shredded and pellets.

Orthopaedic pillows exist in several different shapes and materials. Some promise to keep their shape or mould and conform to your head and shoulders, always keeping spine alignment as the number one focus. Bear in mind, though, that just because a pillow is orthopaedic, doesn't mean it will be good or right for you.

If you are thinking about buying an orthopaedic pillow, consider the different materials they are made from, and pull them out of their boxes and inspect them before you buy. Read the labels to understand what you are purchasing and what the promises are. It's also a good idea to consult a physiotherapist about the best position to use them in as I've seen a number of my clients aggravate neck or shoulder pain after sleeping with an orthopaedic pillow in the wrong position.

Pillows with sponge-type foam that recoils often fall under the same category as orthopaedic pillows. Known for how well they retain their shape, they are often unconventionally shaped.

Husk and seed pillows will also mould to the contours of your head and shoulders and keep the shape until you move. They do have a small disadvantage that no other pillow has, and that is their noise factor. Some people claim that they make a small rustling noise that can be unsettling. The noise is slight, and for many the comfort they offer far outweighs any small sounds the pillows may emit when in use.

Pillow Shapes and Sizes

Contour pillow: A pillow with a curved design that adapts to head, neck and shoulder contour for back sleepers and side sleepers, and can help relieve neck pain and stiffness, frozen shoulder and headaches. Try to buy one that has a flat bit at the back so it doesn't force your neck too far forwards.

Neck pillow or travel pillow: These pillows are horseshoe-shaped, designed for the neck contour. They are called travel pillows since they are mostly used by travellers to keep their neck straight while they take a comfortable nap on board a train or plane.

Wedge pillow: A triangle-shaped pillow that provides a slope for placing the body in a diagonal position. This is a multi-purpose pillow, but is mainly used to relieve the symptoms of acid reflux during sleep.

Lumbar pillow: A half-moon-shaped pillow used at the lower back to comfort and relieve lumbar pain and maintain a correct sitting position. Likewise, they are used underneath knees for leg elevation and as a neck support for relaxation and massage.

Knee pillow: An hourglass-shaped pillow that can be placed between your legs to elevate your lower body and keep a straight side-sleeping position.

Body pillow: A long, curved pillow for total body support that cradles head, neck, shoulders, back, lower back, legs and knees. It replaces other pillows and gives full comfort to the side sleeper.

Gadget pillows: These pillows contain a number of gadgets such as MP3 players to lull you to sleep with calming music; fragrance pillows to calm you with soothing smells; chill pillows to help cool you down and so on. If you want to buy these pillows don't let the promise of a gadget compromise on the comfort.

Gill, 45, had been experiencing chronic neck pain following a road traffic accident three years previously in which she sustained a whiplash injury. She was unable to get off to sleep at night without the use of painkillers. Gill likes to sleep on her right side and is a petite lady with a narrow frame. The gap between her shoulder and neck was small, but all the pillows she had been buying were designed for 'Mrs Average'. I showed her how to 'butterfly' the pillow so that it fitted her neck and allowed her neck to be in the midline position to reduce pain.

HOW TO MAKE A BUTTERFLY PILLOW

Tie a soft scarf, hair band, string, elastic or bandage around the middle of the pillow to make it form a butterfly shape. Put your head on the narrowed part of the pillow and tuck the edges around you. Many patients find a butterfly pillow reduces pain.

By providing yourself with comfortable pillows on a regular basis, that goal of a full night of restful sleep will not be just a dream. I also suggest that once you find that pillow of your dreams you try and see if there are any smaller travel versions of it available so that you can take it with you when you are sleeping away from home.

BED LINEN

Before you head out to purchase bed linen, ask yourself: 'Just what do I like to feel on my skin when I climb into bed? Do I prefer soft and cool, crisp and cool or warm?' Once you have considered your comfort preferences, you are ready to investigate the many fabrics that sheets are made of. The most popular bed sheets are cotton, linen and polyester. The quality of the fabric you buy is determined by the number of threads woven per inch – the higher the number the better the quality of the material.

Most people prefer cotton for bed sheets because it is long-lasting, comfortable, absorbent and suitable for any climate. Silk sheets are luxuriously soft and deliciously comforting and warm in winter, and best at preventing skin creasing. The downside is that they are quite expensive and not so durable, and they can also cause a lot of sliding around the bed at night.

Perhaps the healthiest choice of bed sheet is linen. Linen does not become as soiled as cotton, or absorb as much moisture. It is ideal for hot climates or in the summer because it is light and cool. Although expensive, linen sheets are also extremely long-lasting; two sets could easily last 10 years.

When choosing your bed sheets opt for colours that you find relaxing. White and pastel shades tend to be best. Avoid dark, bright colours, designs and stripes as they can be less restful to the eye. Although you can't see the colour or design of your bed linen during the night, it is important for your bedroom to look as calm, peaceful and relaxing as possible (*see Chapter 6*).

DUVETS

The weight, softness and warmth of a duvet depend on its tog rating and filling. Tog ratings are based on a duvet's ability to trap warm air. Natural-filled duvets have better thermal properties than synthetic ones, and need less filling to achieve the same level of warmth, so their weight can be deceptive. You just need to remember that the higher the tog rating, the warmer the duvet:

➤ Lightweight summer duvet 3.0–4.5 tog
➤ Spring/autumn weight duvet 7.0–10.5 tog
➤ Winter weight duvet 12.0–13.5 tog

Duvets containing feather and/or down are also given a 'fill power'. This is the volume occupied by the filling and it varies depending on the quality. It's about how well the filling recovers and relates to thermal efficiency. The higher the fill power, the better the duvet.

If you don't want to buy a winter and a summer duvet, go for medium tog strength and add a warm blanket in the winter. Blankets may seem a little old-fashioned these days but many of my clients use them, and I always use blankets over my duvet during the cold winter months. The one kind of blanket I don't recommend for regular use is electric blankets, as these may be linked to an increased risk of poor health, infertility and cancer.

Natural duvet fillings are made from duck down or the

superior goose down, or a combination of both. The benefit of natural fillings is that they allow your skin to breathe. Synthetic fillings offer a more practical duvet. Unlike natural duvets that should be professionally cleaned, synthetic ones can be washed in a domestic washing machine – handy if they need to be cleaned regularly.

Technology nowadays means that synthetic duvets are better than ever. They give just as much warmth as feather-filled duvets. Fillings will normally be made from polyester, or with polyester microfibre – a specially light and fine polyester fibre that's air-blown into the duvet casing for good tog and softness. It's designed to emulate the characteristics and feel of down. These duvets are generally a little more expensive than those made of other types of polyester but the feel of the duvet is extra soft and especially cosy.

If you like your bed to have a fuller, well-made look, or find that you and your partner tend to fight over the duvet, then you might want to choose one that's a size larger than your bed or to have single duvets each.

CARING FOR YOUR DUVET

Keep your duvet inside a duvet cover so it stays clean and fresh. You should also try to shake and fluff the duvet every morning after use. As far as washing goes, duvets used inside duvet covers rarely need to be laundered. Instead, wash the duvet cover frequently. If you do need to wash your duvet make sure you use a gentle heat in the dryer then remove and adjust the duvet so damp areas are exposed before returning it to the dryer for another cycle. Hang the duvet out to air-dry for at least 24 hours to make certain all sections are dry before replacing on the bed. Very large duvets may need to be laundered or dry-cleaned commercially since their volume is more than most home washers can handle.

WHAT TO WEAR IN BED

Sandy, *44, was always freezing when she got into bed and didn't give herself time to warm up under the duvet. She wore a vest, sweatshirt, knickers, tracksuit bottoms and socks under the duvet and blanket. Without fail, she would wake overheated at 2am and strip off to her knickers so that she could continue her sleep.*

Your choice of nightwear may be affecting the quality of your sleep. At night time you need to wear loose-fitting, comfortable garments that breathe – cotton is highly recommended. When buying nightwear the key should always be comfort rather than style, so choose something that moves with you properly during sleep, even if it is a size bigger than you wear during the day.

Keeping your neck and shoulders warm is most important, which is why I don't recommend sleeping in skimpy negligees. After making love it's a good idea to get changed into something warmer so you don't wake up with neck ache or stiffness in the morning.

When buying night clothes explore your many choices, including short and long gowns, fancy lingerie, boxers and a T-shirt, and pyjamas (with either short or long legs and sleeves) and then consider all the variables: Do you turn off the heat at night? Sleep under a heavy quilt? Open your window? Use the air conditioner? Dress accordingly if you prefer to be warm, very warm, cool or downright chilly. A sleeping partner will make the bed even warmer and should be counted as a variable.

Keep in mind that flannel is warmer than cotton, and cotton will keep you cooler than silk or polyester. And unless it is a really hot day (or a hot date) I'm going to urge you to buy and wear a pair of bed socks. Due to the fact that they have the poorest circulation, the feet often feel cold before the rest of the body. A recent study has shown that this boosts your chances of a good night's sleep.

If you are comfortable sleeping naked at home and aren't worried about being seen if you have to get up at night there is no reason why you can't. To reduce the risk of neck pain in the morning from catching a draught, however, it is important to ensure that your neck and shoulders stay warm.

SIX

The Bedroom and Bedtime Routine

Is your bedroom preventing a good night's rest? While your home may be your castle, it is your bedroom that's your personal retreat. It should be a place that welcomes you, relaxes you and reflects your personality. It should be somewhere you look forward to spending time each night and enjoy waking up in the morning. It really is important to associate your bedroom with pleasure and rest, not with stress and tension, because creating the right atmosphere can help you sleep better.

Every single time you walk into your bedroom – whether it is to open a window or go to sleep – you should feel relaxed. The atmosphere should be soothing to you, even on a bad day.

SLEEPING ENVIRONMENT

Design your sleeping environment to establish the conditions you need for sleep – cool, quiet, dark, comfortable and free of interruptions. Select colours that you associate with peace and calm. Many people choose green or blue because it reminds them of the ocean, or pastel shades that are easy and gentle on the eye.

Keep your bedroom free of clutter. Piles of unwashed clothes, bills and other to-dos can create stress and dust. On the other hand, paintings of nature or photographs of loved ones can create a peaceful ambience conducive to rest.

In general, make your bedroom reflect the value you place on sleep, and use it only for sleep and sexual activity, not for watching television, eating, working or surfing the internet. Don't bring your laptop to bed with all the stress and interruptions that come with it.

The only exceptions are soft, gentle music, which can help reduce tension, and reading a book for enjoyment. I've seen music work wonders for the sleeping problems of some of my clients. Sounds affect different people in different ways, so if background music or noise helps you get to sleep this is an option well worth checking out. As always, experiment and find out what works best for you. For example, ocean waves may be relaxing for you but music with the sound of rain may make you want to go to the toilet. Music can also act as white noise, blocking creaking floors and fridges and other sleep-disturbing sounds.

It's probably best to remove televisions and other electrical appliances, such as BlackBerries and phones, from the bedroom. You may be tempted to look at texts or emails from the day; these may prevent you from relaxing and stop you sleeping. Hide illuminated clocks from view or cover them with a cloth to avoid clock-watching at night. A great many people continually look at their bedside clocks at night and then count down the hours they have left to sleep, which can make them anxious.

You may also want to check your bedroom for the following:

TEMPERATURE

The ideal temperature for a good night's sleep hasn't yet been agreed on by sleep experts, and it will differ for everyone, but in general most believe that a slightly cool room contributes to good sleep. Aim for around 16–18°C or 62–65°F, a temperature that matches what occurs deep inside the body when its temperature drops during the night to its lowest level. Research suggests that a hot sleeping environment isn't conducive to a good night's sleep. An air conditioner or fan can help. Generally, temperatures under 12°C or 54°F and over 23°C or 75°F will keep you awake; so make sure your bedroom is cool when you go to bed, but ensure, too, that the heating is on when you wake up, especially if you sleep naked.

HUMIDITY

Some people like to sleep with a window open to allow fresh air to come in but it isn't essential for a good night's sleep, and in some cases it's not advisable as a draught all night can cause neck ache in the morning, and noise levels can disturb sleep. An ideal night-time humidity level for the bedroom is 60–70 per cent. You may want to buy a humidifier, which has an added advantage in that its constant 'white noise' humming may drown out other noises that can disrupt sleep. Clues like waking with a sore throat, dryness in your nose or even a nose bleed are signs of too dry an atmosphere. Placing a bowl of water in your room may therefore be helpful. Some of my clients have found that boiling a kettle in their room before they go to sleep helps.

If you have a computer in your bedroom it will dry out the atmosphere, so it is extremely important to make sure your bedroom has the correct humidity. Having plants in your bedroom during the day and then taking them out at night can also help. Eco-friendly houseplants can help to purify the air.

LIGHT AND DARK

Strong light, like sunlight, is the most powerful regulator of our biological clock, which influences when we feel sleepy and when we are alert. In recent years scientists have discovered that natural daylight has the greatest effect on our sleeping patterns. Daylight also inhibits the night-time secretion of melatonin, the hormone that signals the onset of darkness and the need to sleep.

Street and industrial lighting, bright lights in bedrooms or halls, and lights from television screens, mobiles and computers can make you feel more alert and less sleepy. Some people like to use coloured lighting, and in general warmer colours tend to be associated with sunset and cooler colours with dawn. If the lighting is harsh, a solution could be as simple as putting a different cover on the light or changing lampshades.

About 20 per cent of light can still get through your eyelids when your eyes are shut so, unless you have no problems sleeping in a lighter room, you need to keep your bedroom as dark as you can. Consider using light-blocking shades, lined curtains or even an eye mask so light doesn't interfere with your passage to slumber. If you've had a better night's sleep in a darkened hotel room it may be time to get more effective blinds for your bedroom at home. You may also want to plug in a nightlight so that if you need to go to the toilet during the night you don't expose yourself to bright light.

If you want to wear an eye mask make sure you find one that is comfortable and effective for you. There is a huge range available today. Some fit over your eyes and some above if you don't like the pressure on your eyelids and lashes, so shop around until you find the best eye mask for you.

The amount of exposure you get to light during the day may also be interfering with your sleep. Studies have shown there is a link between light exposure and sleep because higher light levels during the day help regulate the biological clock.

Therefore, at least 30 minutes' exposure to daylight every day is advised. If you find yourself waking earlier than you'd like, why not try increasing your exposure to bright light in the evening? If sunlight isn't available, consider a light box (or light visor), available from specialist retailers.

NOISE CONTROL

Sounds louder than 45 decibels can wake you up – that's the same as someone talking quietly – but even sounds as low as 20 decibels can stop you falling asleep. Make sure that the room is quiet. Running a fan or a 'white noise maker' can help drown out sounds from the outdoors. Interestingly, however, the absence of a familiar noise can also disrupt sleep.

Studies have shown that noise from traffic and aeroplanes can increase the time it takes to sleep. If you find your sleep disrupted by noises such as the screech of sirens, the rumble of trains, the rise and fall of conversation, aeroplanes overhead, a dog barking or a partner snoring (*see Chapter 14*), consider buying ear-plugs.

Ear canals are very much like fingerprints in that no two are alike. So if you want to use ear-plugs the best thing is to experiment with several different brands to establish which are most comfortable. A foam ear-plug that is too big will be very uncomfortable and the protection will be handicapped because the foam will not have had room to expand and mould itself into the ear canal. A plug that is too small will be comfortable but may be loose in the ear, and again the protection will be reduced.

Foam ear-plugs are inserted by rolling the plug between two fingers to squash the foam into a thin tube, inserting into the ear and then holding until the foam has fully expanded. The right size ear-plug inserted properly will be comfortable for a full night's sleep and should be able to lessen distracting noises such as snoring and car alarms. Ear-plugs must be regularly replaced or cleaned thoroughly every morning because as you wear them they become saturated with moisture, ear wax and bacteria. Not only are used plugs unhygienic, they also lose their ability to protect your ears.

Another option to consider is bespoke ear-plugs where you get a mould made of your ear to ensure optimum comfort. Some ear-plugs come with eye masks attached so you get both sound and light protection.

SMELL

A clean bedroom should smell fresh but that should be the result of a clean room and free air rather than overpowering artificial room scents. Filling the bedroom with the right scents at the right times will create the proper atmosphere for relaxation, sleep or romance. The sense of smell is, after all, very powerful – a fragrance can send messages to your brain that evoke vivid images, memories and emotions.

Some natural scents relax you and prepare you for sleep, but do bear in mind that just because a smell is natural it doesn't mean it can't trigger allergies. Aromatherapy oils can help strengthen the association between bedroom and sleep. Oils such as lavender and rose have a relaxing, sedative effect. Sandalwood has a woody, exotic scent that is warming and relaxing. Marjoram has a warm, spicy scent (similar to mild oregano) and is noted for its soothing, warming effects. Sage has an exotic scent, which some people find relaxing. If you use these oils regularly in your bedroom, you will learn to associate the smells with sleep; so when you smell the same fragrances on subsequent evenings, your mind will 'recognise' that it's time for sleep. Please be considerate, though, to any pregnant partners.

There are many different methods for using aromatherapy oils:

Vaporisers/oil burners are popular and readily available, usually made of ceramic or metal. A few drops are placed in a bowl and a tea candle is lit underneath, causing the oil to heat up and evaporate.

A nebulising diffuser is one of the best methods available. It has the advantage of not using a naked flame to generate heat, providing more efficient and prolonged use of your oils. This type of vaporisation is a good choice for larger areas and overnight use.

Fragrance rings are an easy and cheap way of using aromatherapy oils. They hold a few drops of oil and are placed on top of a light bulb. After sitting on the bulb, they become very hot, so be sure to turn off your light and allow the ring to cool down before removing. Gently wiping your light bulbs with a thin coat of perfumed oil can also send calming or sensual scents throughout the bedroom.

A plant sprayer or atomiser may also be used to disperse fragrance into a room. Place four drops of aromatherapy oil into 250ml (9fl oz) warm water and pour into a sprayer. Shake the container well and spray. Avoid spraying over wooden furniture, suede or absorbent fabrics.

You could also use **an aromatherapy eye pillow or wheat bag**, or place a few drops on your pillow or bedding.

EVALUATE YOUR BEDROOM

The way your furniture is placed in your bedroom will affect the way you sleep. For example, if you are facing the door, light from the landing can be disturbing; or if there is a bookcase next to your bed the contents can increase feelings of stress, especially if you store bills or work files there.

According to Feng Shui specialists, if you sleep with your feet facing the door, this is taxing for the body. They also recommend that mirrors should be covered. Many Feng Shui guidelines make great sense, such as removing the television from the bedroom and clearing the bedroom of clutter. Perhaps the best way to make sure your bedroom is conducive to a good night's sleep is to use your common sense and find out what feels right for your personal situation. Take a look at your bedroom. How does it feel to you when you go in? Is it a relaxing place for you or do you feel stress when you enter? Evaluate your bedroom for the following:

➤ Not too cluttered and not too bare for your taste.
➤ Soothing colours and décor: yellow, green, blue and pink are excellent shades for bedrooms.
➤ Comfortable bedding, mattress, pillows.
➤ Colours used for bedding – are they comforting and soothing?
➤ Air quality, humidity and temperature.
➤ Lighting: artificial light sources should be soothing. Out-side light should be easily controlled by blinds or drapes.
➤ Noise and disturbances – are there sources of noise inside the bedroom, nearby or outside?

You should be perfectly comfortable when you go to bed. If you aren't, make the necessary changes. Your bedroom is a retreat for you – and your partner if you are in a relationship – and you should be able to relax and switch off the moment you enter it and shut the door behind you.

SLEEPING AWAY FROM HOME

The same principles apply when you need to stay in a hotel or in someone else's home. You can maximise your chances of a good night's sleep by organising the following:

➤ Reserve a room on a high floor if possible, avoiding rooms at street level. You can also request that your room is not close to lifts, stairwells, vending machines or hospitality suites. If you have to, use the air conditioner fan to mask the noise.

➤ Ask for your room to have an eastern or southern exposure so you are more likely to get the morning sun and to feel alert in the morning; if you don't like the location of your room ask for a change before you unpack.

➤ Keep the room temperature at 18°C or 65°F during the night.

➤ Pack your pillow, eye mask and ear-plugs if you use them. You may also want to request extra pillows and blankets when you check in.

➤ Pack a night light that you can plug in at night if you need to go to the bathroom so you don't expose yourself to bright light.

➤ Shut the ensuite bathroom door to prevent unwanted light, smells and noise disturbing you.

➤ Do any work that you need to do at a desk and not on your bed; the same applies to making phone calls and using your computer.

➤ Unless you have crossed a time zone try to go to bed and wake up at roughly the same time as you would at home.

BEDTIME ROUTINE

When you were a child the chances are your parents established a very clear bedtime routine for you. They may have given you a warm bath, and then settled you in bed with a book to read or have read a book to you, and this helped you drift off to sleep. A routine worked then and it can help you now.

A bedtime routine could be the key to a good night's sleep but as no set routine works for everyone the secret is to find what works best for you. The pointers here are all designed to help you drift off to sleep feeling comfortable and secure.

ROUTINE MATTERS

A regular bedtime routine is essential for creating good sleep habits. The routine should be calm and gentle. Ideally you should try to go to bed at the same time each night but that isn't always possible or practical. The key is to teach yourself to fall asleep whenever you do get to bed, and to establish a progression of thought that will allow you to fall asleep. Most important, the routine should be as consistent as you can make it. Your sleep-time routine might include the following:

➤ **Wind down:** Half an hour before you go to bed avoid exciting television programmes, video games or fierce debates as this will be too stimulating. Sending e-mails and surfing the net should have a cut-off point as well. Keep things as gentle, friendly and calm as possible. Reading a book or a magazine is fine as is writing in a journal, listening to gentle music, doing some tidying up or chatting to (not arguing with) loved ones or friends, preferably in person. It really is important never to go to bed after an argument as stress hormones can interfere with sleep hormones and make it impossible to get a good night's sleep.

➤ **Take it easy:** Some gentle stretching or yoga exercises before bedtime can calm and relax body and mind but don't do anything vigorous. Regular exercise is a helpful tool against insomnia, but not within three hours of bedtime. Exercise is energising and raises your body temperature. Try to arrange your workout either in the morning or at lunchtime. Exercising later than this (unless it's for sex) may disturb your sleep.

➤ **Have a warm bath:** One of the best ways to avoid end-of-the-day anxiety is to take a warm bath before going to bed. This will send the blood away from your brain to your skin surface and make you feel both relaxed and drowsy. Your body temperature, which has been raised by the warm water, will also go down as soon as you enter the relatively cool bedroom, and this will initiate sleepiness. Don't make the water too hot. A hot bath will keep your body temperature raised, making you feel hot and uncomfortable.

➤ **Make love:** The only exception to the no exertion or stimulation rule before bedtime is sex. Researchers have found that satisfying sex, either through masturbation or with a partner, can encourage a better night's sleep. Endorphins – feel-good chemicals – are also released during sex.

➤ **Have a bedtime mantra:** Before you enter your bedroom, take a deep breath. Leave your stress outside the door. Mentally prepare yourself to go in there and sleep. This will take just a few moments but it is essential to walk into your bedroom ready to sleep and expecting to fall asleep easily.

Stick to your routine as much as possible. It doesn't need to be complicated or take a lot of time. In fact, the simpler it is the better. For instance, you may want to develop a simple routine of taking a bath, listening to calming music, drinking a cup of herbal tea and turning the lights out. Or you may find that drinking a cup of warm milk while you do some light reading, or preparing yourself a light snack, helps put you in the state of mind for sleep. (*See Chapter 12 for more about snooze foods.*) Or you may find that once you are in bed a few deep breaths are enough to help you drift off. What's important is to develop a routine that you enjoy and that fits into your lifestyle and then try hard to follow it every night.

Just as you shouldn't rush your bedtime routine you shouldn't try to rush the falling-asleep process. It should take between five and twenty minutes to fall asleep; if you fall asleep too quickly – when your head hits the pillow – this is a sign of sleep deprivation.

There will be nights when your bedtime routine isn't working and you are still wide awake. If this is the case the best advice is to stop trying so hard. If you are not sleepy after half an hour, or if you wake up in the night and can't get back to sleep, get out of bed until you feel drowsy again. Try to stay in the dark or in surroundings that are dimly lit and do some light reading or a repetitive task that doesn't require a lot of brain work, like light housework. The chances are it won't take long before you feel sleepy and want to go back to bed.

SEVEN

Sleeping Positions

Just as there is good standing posture, there is also good sleeping posture. As a physiotherapist I have seen at first hand how the position you sleep in can make the difference between a good and a bad night's sleep. Below are a variety of sleeping postures and my suggestions for adapting these postures to optimise your chances of a restful night's sleep.

MIDLINE POSITION

Some of us may feel comfortable in one position only, while others may choose to sleep in a number of positions. Whichever position is preferred, I recommend keeping the body in the midline. This means maintaining the natural curves of the spine to minimise stresses and strains.

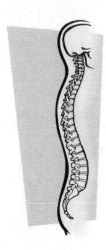

SLEEPING ON YOUR SIDE

Sleeping sideways, stretched out or curled into a foetal position, is the most common sleeping position. Try to avoid sleeping on your arms as this might trigger an attack of pins and needles.

Care should be taken when lying on your side, especially if the mattress is soft and/or you have an hourglass figure. Sinking into the bed may cause an asymmetrical strain on the lower back.

To achieve the midline position, a pillow placed between bent knees will support the hips. If your bed is very soft, pillows can also be placed under the waist or side of your body to support your midriff and back. Make sure your neck is supported by a well-positioned pillow or you could wake up with a headache or a stiff neck. When you are in this position it is most important to make sure you sleep with a straight back, even if you move your feet closer to your body.

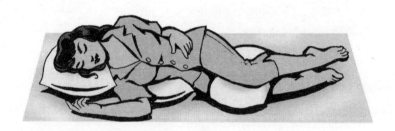

SLEEPING ON YOUR BACK

Sleeping flat on your back may arch it and force your spine into an unnatural position. This can strain your muscles, joints, ligaments, tendons, discs and nerves. Your spine isn't meant to be straight. It has three natural curves: one in your lower back, one in the middle of your back and one near your neck.

To achieve the midline position, place a pillow under your knees to maintain the natural curve of your body and off-load the low back. You should also try to make sure that there are enough pillows to support your neck and head in the midline position, so that they don't tilt forwards or back. If you are a snorer, bear in mind that sleeping on your back can make things worse, but elevating your head can reduce snoring.

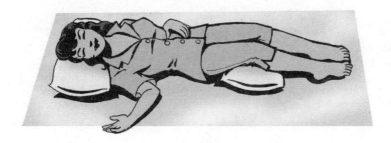

SLEEPING ON YOUR TUMMY

There are people who love to sleep in this position. However, it has the potential to cause the most problems since it exaggerates the arch at the base of your spine. This causes strain on your lower back as well as making your neck turn to one side, causing an asymmetrical strain on your neck. If you must sleep in this position be sure to:

➤ Keep your neck as near to the midline as possible – don't bend it too far forwards or backwards or twist it to one side.
➤ Place a pillow under your tummy and get rid of your head pillow. A pillow can be placed under your chest to minimise neck rotation.

➤ If possible adopt a 'quarter turn' position by slightly raising one side of your body and placing a pillow under your belly to support you, so that you are not lying flat on your stomach.

➤ If you tend to place your hands around your pillow and turn to one side be aware that this will further rotate the neck and predispose you to neck pain.

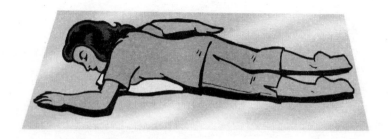

SLEEPING POSITION FOR BACK PAIN

While there are a couple of recommended sleeping positions for back pain sufferers, the best by far is to sleep on your side with your knees bent. If you want, you can use a pillow to support your neck and even put a pillow between your knees.

Some clients find that if they have pain on one side of the back, sleeping on one side may ease the pain while sleeping on the other side may well aggravate it. Try both sides to find out which one works for you.

You may also sleep on your back with a pillow under your knees, and possibly a small pillow under your lower back for support. Sleeping on your stomach is not recommended unless a pillow is used under the hips for support.

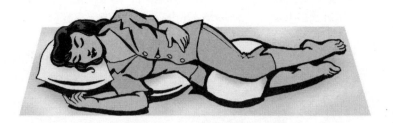

***Clare**, 36, had been waking up with a stiff back ever since the birth of her second child. It took her several hours to get going. When I did a home visit and saw her bed and pillow set-up, I advised her to make some changes. Clare liked to sleep on her back but was aware of an arch in her lower back which became exaggerated in this position. I advised her to place a pillow under her knees to lessen the arch, and to try sleeping on her side in the foetal position. Sleeping on her side took some getting used to but over the next three weeks Clare's back pain reduced and getting going in the mornings wasn't a problem any more.*

GETTING OUT OF BED

It can take a while for joints, muscles, ligaments, tendons and discs to get going in the morning as they have been stationary for several hours while you sleep, so take it easy when you first get out of bed. Spinal discs are full of fluid first thing in the morning, which explains why you are a little taller in the morning than in the evening. This is the time when you are most vulnerable to injury, so avoid strenuous exercise first thing.

To protect your back when getting out of bed, roll onto your side, bend your knees, push your hands to raise yourself up and lower your legs over the side of the bed.

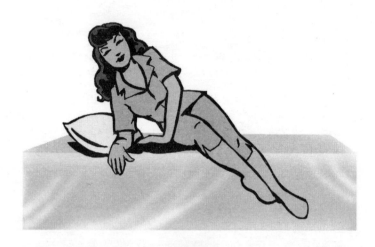

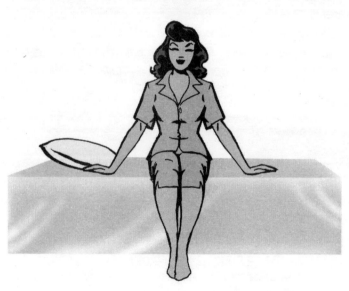

CONTROL YOUR POSITION

You may think that it's impossible to control or change the position you sleep in since you aren't fully aware of what you are doing and you will naturally shift positions in the night. However, it is possible and can make a big difference. When you go to sleep, or when you wake up in the middle of the night, make a conscious effort to return your body to the mid-line by following the above guidelines until they become habitual.

And if you're used to a certain position but that position isn't maximising your chances of a good night's sleep it's time to get out of your comfort zone and try something different. It could make all the difference, but you won't know that until you give it a try.

EIGHT

The Power of Napping

Our culture generally frowns upon daytime sleep. However, many people experience a natural increase in drowsiness in the afternoon, about eight hours after waking. It seems that this post-lunch dip is actually a normal part of the body's circadian rhythm.

Several lines of evidence – including the universal tendency of toddlers and the elderly to nap in the afternoon, and the afternoon nap of siesta cultures – have led sleep researchers to the same conclusion: nature intended us to take a nap in the middle of the day. This biological readiness to fall asleep mid-afternoon coincides with a slight drop in body temperature and occurs whether we eat lunch or not. It is present even in good sleepers who are well rested. Sleep researchers have also discovered that the afternoon dip in mood and alertness is associated with poorer performance, particularly after a night of sleep loss, and a simultaneous increase in sleepiness.

WHY POWER NAP?

Research shows that you can make yourself more alert, reduce stress and improve cognitive functioning with a nap.

Napping may have been part of an evolutionary mechanism to get us out of the hot midday sun. However, because the urge for a nap is appreciably weaker than the need to sleep at night, it can be suppressed (or masked by caffeine) but at the cost of increased sleepiness and reduced mood and performance. Also, because naps conflict with work schedules, they are becoming less common in industrialised societies.

NAPPING IS GOOD FOR BUSINESS

There is a tremendous amount of research – from NASA to the National Sleep Foundation – that supports the notion that a 20-minute daytime nap can rejuvenate people. It improves memory, learning and mood and can boost productivity by up to 30 per cent. Studies have shown that napping is a proven way to clear out the cobwebs and pave the way for a more productive afternoon and evening, whether it's Wednesday or the weekend. A well-timed nap can greatly improve your ability to pay close attention to detail and make critical decisions. In today's hectic world, as our lives become busier and the amount of sleep we get at night is reduced, getting some shut-eye come mid-afternoon could well be one of our most powerful alertness strategies.

INEMURI

A 20-minute nap can boost your work performance far better than a coffee, but pumping your body with caffeine is still considered far more acceptable than resting your head on the keyboard. It's a different story in Japan, however, where dozing anywhere from parliament to business meetings isn't just allowed – it's a sign of how committed you are to your job. It's called *inemuri*, which literally means 'to be asleep while present'. Inemuri is viewed as a sign of exhaustion from working hard and often considered a badge of honour. Some people even fake it to look dedicated to their career.

Strict unwritten rules apply to inemuri, including who can do it – only those high up or low down in a company – and how to do it: it is important to remain upright to show you are still socially engaged in some way. There are even special napping pillows of different shapes and fragrances so that optimal body positioning can be achieved whilst napping.

The concept of inemuri seems bizarre in the UK but given the proven benefits of napping, the Japanese could be the ones who are getting it right. And as for it being a sign of working hard, surely it has to be healthier than drowning in coffee to stay awake or sending an e-mail after hours to prove how late you've been working.

HOW LONG SHOULD I NAP?

As Chapter 2 explained, sleep comes in several stages. If your nap takes you from the first stage of sleep (just drifting off) to the second stage (brain activity slows), you will wake up feeling energised and more alert. If your nap takes you into the third and fourth stages (deep sleep), you will not wake easily and will feel groggy and tired.

The first stage of sleep typically lasts for about 10 minutes, and the second stage lasts for another 10 minutes. That makes the 20-minute nap ideal for most people. Naps shorter than 20 minutes may not be as beneficial, and naps longer than 20 minutes can make it more difficult to fall asleep at night, especially if your sleep deficit is relatively small. However, some research has shown that a one-hour nap can have significant restorative effects including a much greater improvement in cognitive functioning. The key to taking a longer nap is to get a sense of how long your sleep cycles are, and try to wake at the end of a sleep cycle. This is because it's actually the interruption of the sleep cycle that makes you groggy, rather than the deeper states of sleep.

As there are pros and cons to each length of sleep, you may want to let your schedule decide: if you have only 20 minutes to spare, take them! But if you could work in an hour's nap, you may do well to complete a whole sleep cycle, even if it means less sleep at night. If you only have five minutes to spare, just close your eyes; even a brief rest has the benefit of reducing stress and helping you relax a little, which can give you more energy to complete the tasks of your day.

TIME TO NAP

The Nano Nap: 10–20 seconds. Sleep studies haven't yet concluded whether there are benefits to these brief intervals, like when you nod off on someone's shoulder on the train.

The Micro Nap: 2–5 minutes. Shown to be surprisingly effective at shedding sleepiness.

The Mini Nap: 5–15 minutes. This nap increases alertness, stamina, motor learning and performance.

The Power Nap: 20 minutes. Includes the benefits of the micro and the mini, but additionally improves muscle memory and clears the brain of useless built-up information, which helps with long-term memory (remembering facts, events and names).

WHO'S GOT TIME?

'I haven't got time to nap' is a common excuse among those who don't nap but everyone has time to nap, however busy they are. If you spend 10 minutes at the coffee machine in the afternoon, why not just find a quiet place and take a 10-minute mini nap instead? So before you assume that napping can't fit into your busy life, take some time to review your schedule, performance and productivity.

Simon, a 38-year-old insolvency practitioner, never really sleeps for more than four or five hours a night. Every so often he has an eight-hour catch-up night. Dynamic, bright, intelligent and focused, Simon is one of those people whom you know is going to be successful. When asked how he manages to stay on top of his game he says, 'I nap. I just pop home (fortunately home is near work), lie down for 20 or so minutes, switch my brain off and then my internal alarm wakes me up to carry on. Initially I feel a bit groggy but quite soon after I feel refreshed and revived, ready to face my next challenge.' I once asked him if he ever feels exhausted. He replied, 'I haven't got the time to feel exhausted!'

Don't feel that you have to nap. Naps should be avoided if you are getting enough sleep at night and don't feel tired during the day. If, however, you feel tired in the afternoon and have a dip in alertness this is a sign that you would benefit from a nap. In general, larks – or early risers – tend to benefit more from naps than owls or those who like to burn the midnight oil.

HOW TO NAP EFFECTIVELY

If you want to obtain more sleep, and the health benefits that go with getting enough sleep, here are some tips for more effective napping and sleeping at night:

➤ Prime nap time is from 1–3pm when your energy level dips due to a rise in the hormone melatonin at that time of day.

➤ Use an eye mask to provide daytime darkness and make your nap more effective. You may also want to wear your ear-plugs and use relaxation tapes.

➤ Avoid caffeine after 10am or it may be hard for you to nap.

➤ Napping within three hours of bedtime may interfere with night-time sleep.

➤ Ensure that you will not be disturbed for the duration of your nap. Reduce the risk of interruption from things that are under your control, such as beepers, phones, computers and doors.

➤ Your body temperature falls when you sleep, so cover up with a blanket (*see pages 84–5 for more information on napping positions*).

➤ Once you are relaxed and in position to fall asleep, set your alarm for the desired duration, ideally a maximum of 20 minutes.

➤ Create a consistent routine with your nap. You shouldn't just nap once or twice a week; you have to do it on a daily basis or you'll screw up your circadian rhythm.

If you don't have time for a power nap, or don't feel comfortable napping during the day, try simply switching your mind off from the day's activities or day-dreaming. This gives your body a rest and produces slower brain waves similar to sleep.

Place yourself in a comfortable position. Lying down would be great but if this isn't possible rest your head on a table or lie back in a chair with your shoes off. Closing your eyes will shut out some distractions. Take a few slow, deep breaths. Now start counting silently each time you breathe out. Count up from one to four then start again. Keep repeating this procedure until the time is up. The goal is to be doing nothing more. If other thoughts come in, simply accept the fact that you are straying from the instructions and bring yourself gently but firmly back to the counting.

You may feel a little groggy after you wake up from your nap. This is perfectly normal and the feeling should leave you after a few minutes, especially if you have restricted your napping time to 20 minutes. Don't drive or do detailed work for 15 minutes after taking a nap. Give yourself time to re-energise.

NAPPING POSITIONS

As our bodies associate lying down with sleep, approximating the lying down position as much as possible will help you drift off.

If there is no opportunity for you to lie down, at least raise your feet. Make sure your head and limbs are well supported. You may need to have a pillow handy for a comfortable head rest. This will prevent your head dropping onto your chin and falling victim to the familiar 'nap nod' often seen on public transport where people are jerked awake by their head falling forwards.

Choose a roll pillow, possibly one that has a built-in pocket for a cool or warm compress. Travel pillows are great if you need to nap on a train, plane or bus. The inflatable ones are convenient because they can be stored flat and inflated with a few breaths. However, some are poorly designed and can cause all kinds of neck aches and strains because they don't fit the contours of your neck properly, so they are best avoided. A more expensive but better choice is a pillow made from heat-sensitive foam which will fit your neck shape no matter what position you are in, sitting or lying down.

Alternatively, you can just sit at a desk and put your head down for a few minutes' rest.

DON'T LET DRIBBLING STOP YOU

If you dribble during sleep, don't let this stop you napping. This disorder is fairly common and doesn't suggest serious health problems, although it can interfere with the quality of your nap and your sleep at night. Slumbering on a wet pillowcase can be irritating, and waking up after a nap with a puddle of saliva on your desk where your head lay can be embarrassing.

Dribbling in sleep may occur for many reasons including posture, illness and dental issues but the simplest explanation is simply that you are sleeping with your mouth open and breathing through your mouth rather than your nose and mouth. You also tend to salivate more when you sleep than when you are awake. Typically, dribbling can be controlled with a slight change in sleeping position or in lifestyle habits. For example, there is a link between dribbling, being overweight and alcohol consumption.

The best advice is to follow the sleep hygiene tips in this book and to visit your dentist regularly to sort out any dental issues. Make sure you brush your teeth and gargle with warm water or mouthwash before you nap or go to bed. A light towel on your pillowcase with some standbys ready when you wake up might also be a good idea.

REVEL IN YOUR NAP

The first and last consideration should be psychological. Remember that you are not being lazy; napping will improve performance and make you more alert when you wake up. Get over the guilt. Nap time is important, so carve time out of your lunch hour, or ask your boss or colleagues to approve nap time in your office or workplace.

Talk to your colleagues if there is resistance and ask a sleep expert to come and give a seminar. After all, studies have shown that many top executives take power naps for a few minutes during the day to help them recharge their batteries. Some companies in the UK, US and Japan have quiet rooms just for this purpose! It has been statistically shown that these napping areas provided for workers lead to less sick time, greater productivity, higher work satisfaction and fewer errors, which can lead to a better bottom-line for any organisation.

As you start to give your body plenty of rest (at night and during the day), you will feel more vibrant and be able to concentrate better. Enjoy your nap!

SLEEP AT NIGHT

Finally, while napping is crucial to getting the sleep you need when you're burning the candle at both ends, don't undervalue the sleep you need at night. The amount of sleep each person needs may depend on different factors, such as age and work schedules, but whatever your circumstances never forget that you need a good night's sleep as well.

NINE

Common Aches and Pains
that Interrupt Sleep

There are a number of common physical conditions that may make it difficult for you to enjoy a good night's sleep and to wake up refreshed, and some are more disruptive than others. In this chapter I'll discuss some of the most commonly reported problems and offer some practical solutions.

BACK PAIN

Back pain is one of the most common causes of pain-related sleeplessness. A staggering eight out of ten of us will experience lower back pain at some point in our lives, and the more severe the pain the more sleep disruption occurs.

Today's sedentary lifestyles and poor diets have an adverse effect on posture (in sitting, standing and sleeping) and can lead to weight gain. This means that joints and muscles are overloaded and not worked through their normal length. Moreover, poor core stability due to poor posture and weak abdominal muscles means that coping with day-to-day activities becomes difficult. Sitting, standing, sleeping and bending with a poor posture will result in lower back pain. Sleep disruption from other causes – such as stress, your partner snoring or a poorly supporting pillow to name a few – can make the pain feel worse. So what can be done?

For lower back pain, it is always better to see a physio-therapist sooner rather than later to find out the cause and get some tips on how to take good care of your back. Physiotherapy uses physical approaches to promote, maintain and restore human function and movement through the application of continuously evolving treatment strategies.

A physiotherapist will *assess* your condition, *explain* your problem and *treat* it to provide maximum benefits in a minimum time-frame. They will want to know if back pain is preventing sleep or if you wake in the night and then feel pain. The problem will then be treated using techniques such as:

➤ manual therapy, including spinal mobilisation/manipulation
➤ soft tissue techniques/massage
➤ muscle balance assessment
➤ postural analysis and correction
➤ acupuncture
➤ biomechanical evaluation
➤ work-station advice
➤ a core stability rehabilitation programme

Advice will also be offered on self-care as well as home exercises.

The following tips may offer prevention and relief of back pain.

MATTRESS CHECK

Ensure your mattress is suitable for your situation. If you are sharing a small mattress, you may sleep in awkward, uncomfortable positions because you are being crowded out. The bigger the better. If your mattress is too soft or too old your back may not be getting enough support. A saggy mattress contributes to muscle stiffness and chronic back pain.

PILLOW CHECK

It is important that your pillow supports your neck in the mid-line so make sure you are using the correct pillow for your needs (*see pages 46–54*).

SLEEPING POSITION

Your sleeping position could be making the problem worse. If you lie on your back try using a pillow under your knees, and if you sleep on your side try putting a pillow between your knees.

GETTING OUT OF BED

Your bed should be a height that makes it easy for you to get into and out of it. If it is too low, get a handyman to raise it using blocks of wood/bricks. When getting into bed, sit on the edge, lower your body onto one elbow and shoulder, and draw up your knees and then feet. Reverse the procedure to get out (*see page 76*).

POSTURE

Pay attention to your posture during the day. More and more of us are leading sedentary lives and are required to sit for long periods, so correct sitting posture is important.

When sitting at home or at a friend's house, try to choose a firm-backed chair as opposed to the sloppy sofa. Sit up and use the back rest for support; push your buttocks well into the back of the chair. When sitting in a chair without a back rest, strive to sit up straight. Drop your shoulders down and bring your chest up, as though there is a string coming down from the roof, pulling your chest up.

When sitting at a computer, bring your adjustable chair close to the desk. Make sure that the monitor is situated directly in front of you. Limit laptop use or use a second keyboard and separate the screen from the key board to avoid slumping.

If sitting for a long period of time, it really is important to get up and stretch every 20 minutes. When standing at a counter or in a queue for long periods, you should also make sure you pay attention to your posture.

ANALYSE YOUR FOOTWEAR

Depending on how much walking or running you do, try to replace your shoes frequently. If you run you may need to change your trainers every six to eight months. They are made from soft materials and flatten after repeated use, resulting in poor foot posture, which in turn will cause back problems. If you are a woman, vary the height of your shoes. You don't need to wear flat shoes all the time; just make sure you wear a variety of different heel heights.

BENDING AND LIFTING

Always bend your knees when you need to pick something up or make the bed; don't bend at the waist. If you need to carry heavy documents use a wheelie bag, and if the items are too heavy get someone to help you. If you have a heavy rucksack make sure you use both straps, and if you are travelling buy a suitcase that you can push or pull along.

WRAP UP WARM

Draughts can magnify muscle spasm so wear as many air-trapping layers as possible. Bear in mind, too, that stress can also increase muscle spasm, so try to watch your stress levels.

BACK STRENGTHENING EXERCISES

It is important to do some core stability work to lengthen and strengthen your trunk muscles as well as to pay attention to the balance and coordination of this area. Keep your pelvic floor and abdominal muscles strong because they support your lower back. A tailored weight-training, ball work and stretching exercise programme will increase muscle tone and help make your back healthier.

Make sure you consult a physiotherapist before beginning any exercise programme. He or she can teach you appropriate exercises and work with you to create a programme that suits your needs.

These stretching exercises can help bring back some suppleness and increase mobility, decreasing back pain and discomfort.

Back flexion exercise: While lying on your back with your knees bent and your feet flat on the floor, gently pull one knee into your chest 10 times, repeat 10 times with the other knee, then 10 times with both knees. To further loosen the lower back, with both knees into your chest, circle your knees 10 times to the right and 10 times to the left. If you feel any pain or discomfort during this exercise, stop.

Hamstring stretches: The hamstrings run through the back of each thigh. Tightness in this muscle limits motion in the pelvis, which can increase stress across the lower back and corrupt correct posture. Stretching the hamstrings can gradually lengthen them and reduce the stress felt in the lower back. To lengthen your hamstrings lie on your back with your knees bent and your feet flat. Interlock your fingers behind your left thigh, pull on the back of your thigh and gently straighten out your lower leg. Hold for 30 seconds and repeat three times. Then repeat on the right side. If you feel any pain or discomfort when stretching your hamstring be sure to stop.

Core stability exercises: Pull your tummy muscles in 100 per cent, and then release 70 per cent, retaining a 30 per cent contraction, and try to maintain this during the day. One way to help you do this is to tie a piece of string around your tummy at a 30 per cent contraction. The string should feel comfortable, not tight. Alternatively, put your belt on the next tightest notch whilst maintaining a 30 per cent contraction. Try doing this for as long as you can.

NECK PAIN

Neck pain, like back pain, is becoming more common due to our increasingly sedentary lifestyles. Getting a good night's sleep when you're suffering from a sore neck isn't easy, and waking up in the morning with a sore neck isn't pleasant. Some people are prone to neck pain because of their occupation; but regardless of how much sitting or bending down you do during the day, you can rid yourself of pain without resorting to anti-inflammatory drugs or painkillers. You need to apply a few tried-and-tested methods, replace bad habits with good ones, and give your neck regular exercise.

GOOD POSTURE THROUGHOUT THE DAY

Keeping your head in an awkward position can cause neck pain. You need to avoid:

➤ craning your neck in front of your shoulders when driving or sitting at the computer screen
➤ turning because your work station is not set up to suit your needs
➤ bending to the side because you are using the phone for long periods or carrying a heavy bag

During the day make a conscious effort to keep your head level, with your shoulders back and down and your chin in, as if a piece of string is pulling the back of your head up. Try to use a document holder at a 45-degree angle when reading documents or a book as this won't stress the muscles in the back of the neck. When sitting, roll up a towel and place it in the small of your back – it will better align your pelvis and lower back and so help with your neck posture.

PUT DOWN THE TELEPHONE

If you talk on the phone a lot, especially while trying to write, you've got your neck in an awkward position – an invitation to stiffness and pain. Try using a speaker phone or headpiece.

HEAT UP AND COOL DOWN

Research is inconclusive but with years of experience as a physiotherapist it seems that personal preferences rule here. I usually recommend heat for pain due to muscle spasm, and ice for pain due to inflammation. However, 80 per cent of my clients prefer heat for all neck ailments. Great heat options include:

➤ microwaveable heat packs
➤ hot water bottles
➤ self-heating stick-on pads
➤ electrical heating pads
➤ hot showers
➤ wrapping up warm

If ice works for you, an ice pack made of frozen peas wrapped in a damp towel is a good choice. Always take care when applying heat and ice to avoid burns.

TAKE A BREAK

Just as your feet need rest from constant standing, your neck needs a break from constant sitting. Your head weighs approximately 3.5 kg (8 pounds), and that's a lot of weight for the neck to support without much help from the rest of your body. So if your job requires you to do a lot of sitting, make sure you stand up and walk around every 20 minutes or so.

EYE LEVEL

If you work with a computer screen all day, it's important to have it positioned at the correct eye level. If you are a touch typist your screen should be slightly above eye level but if you are a 'hunt-pecker' it should be slightly below. To avoid neck strain make sure your work station is set up correctly and your screen is an arm's length away. Ensure that you get your eyes tested annually.

PILLOW TALK

Make sure your pillow supports your neck in the midline. You may want to buy a cervical pillow that gives your neck the right support, but when buying a pillow it is important to find one that is right for you (*see pages 46–54*).

SLEEP ON A FIRM MATTRESS

A lot of neck problems begin, and worsen, with poor sleeping habits. Having a firm mattress is important (*see pages 28–41*).

SLEEPING POSITION

If you sleep on your stomach put a pillow under your chest and tummy and remove the pillow from your head to keep your neck in the midline. Try changing your sleep posture. Sleeping on your side in the foetal position may help (*see page 72*).

WRAP UP

When it's cold and damp outside, make sure you wear a scarf and hat. The weather can aggravate neck stiffness and pain. A draught at night can also cause neck problems, so make sure windows and doors are shut, and the air conditioning isn't too strong. During the day wear polo necks or scarves to ease neck pain. Scarves should be avoided during the night for obvious reasons but do make sure your neck and shoulders are warm.

UNDER PRESSURE?

Just being tense can tighten the muscles in your neck and this can magnify neck pain. If you're under a lot of pressure or feel tense a lot, it can help to learn coping strategies when tension mounts, such as taking time out or listening to gentle music.

EXERCISE AWAY NECK PAIN

Your neck muscles need to be lengthened and strengthened. Here are some exercises to combat stiffness and prevent problems in the future. Do each exercise five times, five times a day. Do the first three exercises for two weeks before starting the rest. **Stop** if you feel any pain or discomfort.

Yes exercise: Slowly tilt your head forwards as far as possible. Then move your head backwards as far as possible.

Maybe exercise: Tilt your head towards your shoulder, while keeping your shoulder stationary. Straighten your head then tilt towards the other shoulder.

No exercise: Slowly turn your head from side to side as far as possible.

After repeating these exercises for two weeks, place your left hand on the left side of your forehead while you push towards the left with your head. Use an equal and opposite force. Hold for five seconds and then relax. Repeat five times. Then do the same exercise on the right.

With your right hand on the front of your forehead push your head forwards. Provide only slight resistance to the front of your head while you push your head forwards. Then push your head backwards with your right hand on the back of your head. Provide only slight resistance to the back of your head while you push your head backwards.

CRAMPING PAIN

Painful night-time leg cramps can wake you up and ruin a perfectly good night's sleep. When cramps wake you, they can linger for half an hour or so and make going back to sleep very difficult indeed. If they happen frequently enough, you can begin to dread bedtime.

When cramps occur during sleep, it's usually because of a magnification of a muscle reflex that happens normally. As you roll over in your sleep, your calf muscles involuntarily contract, and the tendons stretch along with them. Nerve stretch receptors in the tendon come alive and relay a message to the spinal cord instructing the calf muscles to contract, or spasm. You may not be aware of this at times, but at other times the muscles will not relax causing pain.

Other causes of night-time leg cramps can include:

➤ a pinched nerve
➤ muscle damage
➤ mineral deficiencies, particularly potassium and magnesium
➤ diabetes
➤ hormonal fluctuations
➤ peripheral vascular disease
➤ diuretic medication

If you feel any of these may be contributing to your cramps, see your doctor. He or she will examine your general health before probing further into your medical background if necessary.

DEALING WITH CRAMPS

When pain strikes, stretch the contracted muscle and flex your foot. If you are flexible enough, pull your big toe towards you.

You could also try to stand up and straighten out your leg, massaging it to get the blood flowing. The muscle may try to contract again almost instantly so keep it straight and continue to massage it until it goes away. Fortunately, most cramps go away within five or ten minutes, but if your cramping is more prolonged or occurs more than two or three times a week, consult your GP.

CALF STRETCHING EXERCISE

1. Stand about 1 metre (3 feet) from a wall, facing it.
2. Step forwards with your left foot.
3. Put your hands on the wall at chest level. Bend your elbows slightly and aim your shoulders, hips and feet towards the wall.
4. Bend your left knee gently and feel the stretch in your right calf muscle as you do so. Keep both heels on the ground at all times.
5. Hold the stretch for at least 15 seconds.
6. Repeat with the other side.

PREVENTING CRAMPS

Research may not have identified the exact cause of leg cramps but a little prevention can go a long way to improving your nocturnal quality of life. Applying a heat pad to your muscles for 10–15 minutes before sleep can be of assistance. Massaging and stretching your calf muscles before bedtime can also help to exhaust the stretch reflex.

Research suggests that taking a multivitamin and mineral supplement containing potassium, calcium, vitamin E and magnesium – or adding foods to the diet that are rich in these elements – may reduce the incidence of night-time leg cramps. Maintaining your hydration levels is important, especially if you've been exercising vigorously. When you sweat, you lose salts from your body; a sports drink can help to replace the electrolytes lost. Regular exercise and stretching can also help reduce the risk of cramping at night.

PINS AND NEEDLES

Pins and needles (paraesthesia) is a sensation of uncomfortable tingling or prickling, usually felt in the hands or feet. The affected area is sometimes said to have 'fallen asleep'. Waking up in the middle of the night with a painful attack of pins and needles in your arms, hands or legs can interfere with a good night's sleep, not only because it wakes you up but also because it is uncomfortable and distressing and it can take a while to get comfortable and relaxed again.

The best way to deal with pins and needles is to prevent them happening in the first place. A common cause is leaning or lying awkwardly on a limb, which either presses against the nerves or reduces the blood supply to the local area. To prevent this happening, position pillows between your legs or under your arms.

Less commonly, nutritional deficiencies – particularly low calcium levels – can cause pins and needles so make sure your diet is healthy. Excessive amounts of alcohol can also trigger an attack. Pins and needles in the feet can be a sign of nerve damage or poorly controlled diabetes. Recurrent bouts of pins and needles should always be discussed with your doctor as more serious causes include neurological disorders.

DEALING WITH PINS AND NEEDLES

If you do get an attack change your position immediately to restore the blood supply. In some cases, rocking your head from side to side will painlessly remove the sensation in less than a minute. This is because a tingly hand or arm is often the result of compression in the bundle of nerves in the neck, and loosening the neck muscles releases the pressure. Compressed nerves lower in the body govern the feet, and standing up and walking around will typically relieve the sensation. An arm that has fallen asleep may also be woken more quickly by clenching and unclenching the fist several times; the muscle movement increases blood flow and helps the limb return to normal.

RESTLESS LEGS SYNDROME (RLS)

*For the past 10 years **Sonia**, 52, has been experiencing problems falling asleep. She describes a tingling sensation in her legs and feet when she lies down and the uncontrollable urge to kick them. It can take up to four hours for her to fall asleep and she dreads lying down because of this. Her anxiety about not being able to fall asleep has made things worse; the more anxious she becomes the more she needs to move her legs and the longer it takes her to get to sleep.*

This is a form of sleep-related movement disorder and often involves an irresistible desire to move your legs. The sensations may be pain, discomfort, itching, tingling, prickling or ants crawling up your legs. When the legs are moved there is often a relief of this sensation, but symptoms return when the leg movements stop.

Up to 15 per cent of the population suffer from restless

legs syndrome and the peak onset period is middle age. It is more common in women. People who are anaemic are at higher risk, and for this reason iron supplementation may be advised. The syndrome may also be caused by an underlying neurological or medical disorder, such as diabetes, so it is always important to have this ruled out by your doctor if attacks are severe.

DEALING WITH RLS

Simple lifestyle changes, such as walking and stretching, warm baths, massage and relaxation exercises, can help correct the disorder. Studies have also shown that maintaining a regular sleep pattern can reduce symptoms. Some individuals, finding that RLS symptoms are minimised in the early morning, change their sleep patterns. Research suggests that dietary supplementation with iron, folate, magnesium and calcium may also be advised. If none of these strategies help, prescription medication and referral to a sleep movement disorders specialist may be the best solution.

HEADACHES

Research shows that there is a link between sleep disturbances and headaches and migraines, especially with headaches that occur in the night or early evening, although what causes what is not yet known. What we do know, though, is that quality sleep is one of the best ways to prevent the onset of headaches. Unfortunately, getting a good night's sleep when you are prone to headaches or, even worse, migraines, is easier said than done. Not only does lying down make it worse but you are also much more sensitive than usual to noise, light and other disturbances, making it hard to stick to your bedtime routine.

As each person's pattern of headaches or migraines is different, so are the coping techniques for relaxation and sleeping. Some people have success with the non-medication techniques, others need medication to provide relief, and still others need a combination of medication and non-medication techniques.

It's best to avoid over-the-counter painkillers as many contain caffeine which can make sleeping problems worse. The following are tried-and-tested non-medication techniques but if none of them prove effective, make an appointment with your doctor to discuss the options available to you. Whatever you do, don't ignore headaches that occur over and over again. They could be a sign of an underlying health problem, such as undiagnosed high blood pressure or diabetes.

FIND A PATTERN

See if you can find a pattern or a trigger to your headaches and then avoid that trigger. When you get a headache, note what is going on in your life at the time. Are you under stress? Have you been having problems sleeping? Stress and poor quality sleep can trigger headaches so stress management and good sleep hygiene are essential. Other tension headache triggers include too much sleep, lack of exercise, and activities that require repetitive motion such as chewing gum, grinding teeth or staring at something fixed like a computer screen for long periods of time.

LEARN TO RELAX

By reducing muscle tension you may be able to ward off a fair number of headaches. Sit in a dark, quiet room for 20 minutes. Place an ice pack on your forehead. Tension headaches sometimes respond better to the application of heat. Try to regard headaches or migraines as evidence that the body needs time to be alone, to recharge. Lie in total silence, in complete darkness and sleep, if possible, until the headache is gone.

SKIP THE LIE-IN

Snoozing in for more than an hour can disrupt your sleep-wake cycle, and anything that tinkers with your body's natural rhythms may prime you for pain. Commit to waking up (and going to bed) at the same time every day – yes, that includes weekends, too.

WATCH YOUR POSTURE

Are you sitting or standing up straight with your shoulders down and back? If not, readjust. The main sensory nerve in your forehead is rooted in the base of your neck – which is why experiencing muscle tension there or in your shoulders can lead to head pain.

If you use a computer during the day and are a touch typist, your monitor needs to be slightly higher than your eyes, but if you need to look up and down when you type it should be slightly lower.

BED AND PILLOW MOTS

Make sure you are using the correct pillows and mattress as poor sleeping posture can trigger headaches (*see Chapters 4 and 5*).

RAISE YOUR GLASS

Drink plenty of water during the day as dehydration can trigger headaches.

WATCH WHAT YOU EAT

Missing meals or nutrients can trigger headaches so make sure you don't leave more than a few hours between meals and snacks.

Take note of what you have been eating. Watch out especially for foods such as cheese, red wine, chocolate, citrus juice or fruit that contain tyramine, phenylethylamine and histamine, which can all trigger headaches. Unfortunately, symptoms often don't hit you immediately after eating these foods, so you need to keep a diary for several weeks to notice a pattern.

Magnesium helps your muscles to relax and a deficiency can trigger headaches. Current research suggests that eating leafy green vegetables, nuts and seeds, bitter chocolate, soya beans and whole grains may help.

Make sure your diet is rich in essential fatty acids – especially omega 3 found in oily fish, nuts and seeds. Another study suggested that migraine sufferers showed a significant reduction in symptoms when they took omega 3 fish oils every day.

WHEN PAIN STRIKES

If you have a tension headache and can't get to a dark room to relax, put your hands around the back of your head and drop your chin towards your chest. Press your chin down and hold for a minute. Then use your hands to turn your head to the right and hold for a minute; then back to the centre and hold for a minute; then to the left for a minute and then back to the centre, again for a minute. If you find that this exercise worsens your headache, stop immediately. If your hair is long, tying it up in a high bunch can also help ease pain. If your symptoms worsen, loosen your bunch.

PHYSIOTHERAPY

Headaches can be treated with a wide variety of different methods including:

➤ a thorough spinal assessment
➤ manual therapy, including spinal mobilisation/manipulation
➤ soft tissue techniques/massage
➤ muscle balance assessment
➤ postural analysis and correction
➤ acupuncture
➤ biomechanical evaluation
➤ work-station advice
➤ a core stability rehabilitation programme

Advice will also be offered on self-care as well as home exercises.

MASSAGE

Regular exercise and stretching can prevent many tension headaches. Treat yourself to a neck, shoulder and head massage. Whether it is a traditional massage or acupressure, releasing physical tension and improving circulation can promote feelings of wellbeing and even prevent headaches. Simply rubbing your temples can relieve pain.

TAKE A WARM BATH

In some cases a warm bath can make headache sufferers feel better, especially if an essential herb such as lavender is added. Other helpful oils include rosemary, lemon and chamomile, which can stimulate blood supply to the head, and eucalyptus, which eases pain. Add a few drops to your bath or make up a massage oil for the neck and shoulders.

ORGASM

Some people find that orgasm can help get rid of headaches as it opens up the blood vessels. There are no studies to prove this but it's surely worth a try!

ALTERNATIVE THERAPIES

One study showed that 70 per cent of migraine sufferers had less frequent attacks when taking the herb feverfew. The herb milk thistle may also be beneficial as it helps improve liver function. Acupuncture and homeopathy may also help with headache prevention and treatment.

WAKING UP WITH A HEADACHE?

Do you wake up every morning with a headache? You're not alone. A recent study published in *The Archives of Internal Medicine* said that one in thirteen people do, and none of these people had been out drinking the night before. Chronic morning headaches are usually associated with sleep disorders such as sleep apnoea, in which people stop breathing many times throughout the night (*see pages 119–21*), teeth grinding and periodic limb movements. And the bed partners of snorers are known to wake with a headache. But the study found that the headaches were most strongly linked to anxiety and depression. So if you regularly wake up with a morning headache try the prevention tips listed above and the good sleep hygiene and stress-management tips in this book, and if they don't offer relief within two weeks seek advice from your GP.

TEN

Common Ailments that Keep You Awake

SNORING

If your snoring or breathing sounds like a combine harvester or wind machine when you go to sleep then snoring is having a big effect on your sleep, your relationship (if you are in one) and your health.

Mention snoring and most people laugh but the long-term effects of snoring are far from amusing. Snoring is said to disturb the sleep of at least 20 per cent of the adult population and has led to marital breakdowns and even to murder. A recent survey found that 81 per cent of men snored for more than 10 per cent of the night and 22 per cent snored for more than 50 per cent of the night. Other studies have suggested that women who sleep with a snoring partner tend to have more health problems and a poorer quality of sleep. Although research shows that snoring is less common in women, up to 20 per cent do snore and this increases after menopause.

Snoring is a sleep-related breathing disorder caused by vibrations of the tissues behind the nose and mouth. Alcohol, weight gain, sleeping pills, sleep apnoea (*see pages 119–21*) and smoking are all thought to trigger snoring.

Inexplicably, most snorers never wake themselves up with their snores but if a partner or friend can do some taping or videoing, this can sometimes be enough of a shock to spur the snorer on to make changes.

STOP SNORING TIPS

Although there is no universal cure for snoring, if you are at your wits' end with being dug in the back and told to roll over every hour then read my stop snoring tips:

Elevate Your Head

Elevating your head by sleeping on a thicker pillow or multiple pillows will help reduce your snoring. Take care if you have neck or back pain. Sleep on a firmer pillow, as a pillow that's too soft encourages your throat muscles to relax and narrows your air passageway.

Foods and Medicines to Avoid

Don't drink alcoholic beverages or take sleeping pills, tranquillisers or antihistamines just before going to sleep. They will cause your muscles to relax and limit your air passageway.

Don't eat a big meal just before bed. If your stomach is full it will push up on your diaphragm and limit the breathing passageways. Especially avoid eating rich foods such as cakes, biscuits, chocolate and pizza. Also, pass on dairy products just before you go to sleep, as they can cause a build-up of mucus.

Sleep on Your Side

Sleeping on your side instead of your back may help to prevent snoring. If you sleep with your partner, ask them to tell you which side you snore less on; the left or the right. An old-fashioned remedy to prevent sleeping on your back is to sew a tennis ball to the back of your nightwear; the discomfort of sleeping on the ball will prevent you from staying on your back. However, this may lead to a disrupted night and isn't recommended.

Anti-snoring Products

There is a range of anti-snoring products available such as the 'snore stopper', an electronic device that wakes you up when you snore, and anti-snoring nasal spray, which prevents snoring by keeping the nasal path open. If you want to use any of them you will need to experiment to find what works best for you. Bear in mind that some of these products can make your throat feel dry, so make sure you have a bottle of water by your bed.

Other Tips

➤ If you are overweight, losing some weight will reduce snoring by increasing the space in your air passageway.

➤ Follow a regular sleep routine.

➤ Inhale steam before sleeping or sleep in a room with a humidifier turned on to reduce congestion and moisturise the throat.

➤ If you are a smoker, stop smoking before bedtime, or at least just before you go to bed. Smoking causes inflammation and swelling of the throat.

➤ If nasal obstruction is the cause try nasal dilators or strips. Nasal dilators keep your nasal path open, which can reduce snoring. They might look a little odd but they are quite comfortable to wear.

If your snoring continues to adversely affect your sleep and your health, consult a medical professional. They will be able to diagnose or rule out sleep apnoea (*see pages 119–21*) and see what treatments and, if necessary, surgery might help. Bear in mind that there is a link between snoring and obesity so healthy eating and regular exercise to lose weight may also be advised.

WHAT'S CAUSING YOUR SNORING?

The British Snoring and Sleep Apnoea Association (BSSAA) – www.britishsnoring.co.uk – was formed in 1991 to help the 30 million people in the UK whose sleep is disrupted by snoring. It offers information on causes and treatment and the following tests to help identify the cause of your snoring. Once you know where your snoring is originating from, you can find an appropriate treatment to control it.

Nose test: Looking in a mirror, press the side of one nostril to close it. With your mouth closed, breathe in through your other nostril. If the nostril tends to collapse try propping it open with the clean end of a matchstick. If breathing is easier with the nostril propped open, nasal dilators may solve your snoring problem. Test both nostrils. Purchase some nasal strips and put them on before going to sleep. Nasal strips will open up your nostrils and allow more air to come in, thus reducing snoring.

Mouth breathing test: Open your mouth and make a snoring noise. Now close your mouth and try to make the same noise. If you can only snore with your mouth open then you are a 'mouth breather'. A snore guard will help keep your mouth closed and encourage you to breathe correctly through your nose.

Tongue test: Stick your tongue out as far as it will go and grip it between your teeth. Now try and make a snoring noise. If the snoring noise is reduced with your tongue in this forward position then you are probably what is known as a 'tongue base snorer'. The most appropriate control for tongue base snoring is a mandibular advancement device. These range from simple boil and bite dentures to dentist-fitted, self-adjustable devices aimed at moving the jaw forwards.

If none of these make any difference, try doing these tests in different positions such as lying on your front, back and sides with a variety of pillow numbers.

STRESS AND ANXIETY

*For the last six months, **Pam**, 28, found that her sleep was frequently broken by toilet visits, tossing and turning and worrying about the outcome of an impending court case. To escape her daily anxiety, palpitations and sweating, she would have a few hours' sleep in the afternoon. She then felt guilty about her daily kip, which exacerbated her anxiety. She eventually used a diary to plot her daily anxiety patterns and saw a clear connection between a restless night and her daily sleep; she stopped napping and slept much better at night.*

In my work as a physiotherapist I've seen at first hand how stress can cause sleeping problems. Common triggers include job-related pressures; a family, relationship or marriage problem; and a serious illness or death in the family. Usually the sleep problem disappears when the stressful situation passes. However, if short-term sleep problems aren't managed properly from the beginning, they can persist long after the original stress has passed. If you are under stress, take some time to unwind properly before going to bed. Some people find visualisation or deep breathing, or a cup of calming chamomile tea, helpful. If something is troubling you, and there is nothing you can do about it right away, try writing it down before going to bed and then tell yourself to deal with it tomorrow. (*See also bedtime routine, pages 68–70, and dreams, Chapter 16.*)

You need to avoid worries about work and other issues at bedtime. If your mind is too active you won't be able to sleep well and may even wake up in the night with anxious thoughts. So try to calm your mind before going to bed. You may want to make one of the following tension-releasing techniques part of your bedtime routine as you lie in bed with the lights off:

DEEP BREATHING

As you lie in bed take some deep breaths and concentrate only on your breathing. This can help induce relaxation, or you may prefer to add a mantra each time you breathe in such as, 'I'm feeling calm, peaceful and serene. I am falling asleep slowly.'

VISUALISATION

You may want to imagine yourself in a situation where you know you will feel content and happy. Examples are a tropical paradise, sailing on calm waters, walking through fields, flying in the air or feeling the warmth of the sun and hearing the gentle trickle of running water. You could also visualise a flickering candle in front of you. Focus your mind on the candle and watch it until it stops flickering and your mind becomes calm.

THINK BACKWARDS

Try to remember your day backwards. Sounds easy until you try it. Start from your bedtime routine and work your way backwards to when you woke up. You probably won't make it to lunchtime!

COUNT SHEEP

This old technique can work for some people but others may find that counting actually wakes them up so find what works for you. If you want to give it a try it doesn't have to be sheep: you can count cows, hens, horses, chickens or dogs, but you need to make the scene as uninteresting as possible so that you literally bore yourself to sleep.

PROGRESSIVE MUSCLE RELAXATION (PMR)

This is a great way to help you unwind and prepare your body for sleep. As you lie in bed try tensing and relaxing your muscles in groups from your toes right up to your forehead. Squeeze each muscle group for a few seconds then release and relax for 10 seconds before moving on to the next.

1. To begin, think about your toes. Scrunch your toes up and then relax them until you can feel them tingle.
2. Now think about the rest of your feet. Point your feet and then relax them.
3. Think about your calves. Flex or tense them and relax them.
4. Repeat with your thighs, buttocks, abdomen, back and shoulders, arms, hands, fingers, forehead, face and finally your eye muscles.

The first couple of times you use this kind of relaxation technique you may have to get all the way up to the top of your head and start over again at your toes. That's okay. Begin again. The important thing is to feel yourself relax and begin to sleep. A variation on this exercise is simply to raise your hands over your head and have a good stretch, tensing every muscle, even your face. Then with arms still raised, let all the tension relax.

USEFUL TIP

If you're finding it hard to drift off, try closing your eyes and rolling your eyeballs up three times. This happens naturally when you sleep and may help trigger the release of sleep chemicals, such as melatonin.

TEETH GRINDING

Recent research has shown that grinding teeth during sleep (sleep bruxism) affects up to 8 per cent of the population and is associated with stress and other disorders such as sleep apnoea (*see pages 119–21*), headaches (*see pages 101–106*), tooth decay and daytime sleepiness.

Bruxism is more likely to occur in people with sleep apnoea and in people who snore or drink heavily, and to a lesser extent in caffeine drinkers, smokers and people with stressful lifestyles. Treatment includes improving sleep hygiene and the use of a plastic tooth guard or splint during the night. If you don't know if you grind your teeth at night ask your dentist.

ALLERGIES

Do you wake up groggy in the morning or feel fatigued during the day? Perhaps allergies are the culprit. There may be something in your house or in your bedroom that is triggering an allergic reaction that makes it hard for you to sleep. Dust mites and household dust are most common (*see pages 43–44*) but new carpets, new curtains, cleaning sprays, washing powder, air fresheners and fresh paint release chemical emissions that can also cause problems.

Avoidance is always the best treatment for allergies, regardless of which allergens are the triggers. Many people choose medications or vaccinations, despite their drawbacks, and forget that there are lots of simple methods – both old and new – to help with avoidance. The good news is that you really don't have to strip your home down to the bare bones to make it allergy-proof. Thorough and regular cleaning generally makes a huge difference in keeping your home as free of mould and dust as possible. Patients with asthma or allergic rhinitis due to dust mites, mould or other indoor allergens can feel better by keeping their home cool (20–22°C or 68–72°F) and making sure there is good ventilation. Plants in your bedroom during the day but taken out at night can also help absorb dust, as can the use of specially designed allergy pillows.

NIGHT SWEATS

Night sweats can be caused by bouts of stress and anxiety as well as by a bedroom or bedclothes that are too warm. For women, night sweats can also be caused by hormonal changes that occur during peri-menopause, the years of gradual hormonal change prior to menopause, which typically begins in the late 30s and early 40s. Some women suffer only mildly from hot flushes, whereas others find they are hot and soaking even in the cold of winter.

Night sweats and hot flushes feel like sudden waves of heat that strike at any time and any place. They can start at the waist or chest, but generally work their way to the neck and face, causing flushing, blushing, perspiration and discomfort.

Aside from medical interventions there are a number of natural measures you can adopt to ease your discomfort. First of all wear natural fibres such as cotton; these are better able to disperse heat and take it away from the body, helping you feel more cool and relaxed. Silk sheets can also help cool off your sleep environment, as can an open window and extra fan or two.

There are many identifiable triggers that contribute to hot flushes that should be avoided. These include spicy and acidic foods, sugar, hot drinks, alcohol, stress, hot weather, caffeine, saturated fats, smoking and even anger.

Consider having a glass of iced water nearby to help cool you off if you have an attack in the middle of the night. For a portable hot flush remedy, place a few drops of basil or thyme essential oil on a tissue or cotton ball and wrap in clingfilm. Open and inhale for instant relief. You may also want to try using chill pillows, which are designed to help keep you cool during the night. Studies also show that regular exercise and a healthy diet rich in fruit and vegetables, oily fish, nuts, seeds and whole grains, and that includes plenty of phyto-oestrogens (found in soya, legumes, grains and vegetables), can reduce hot flushes significantly.

MEDICATIONS

Bear in mind that certain medications such as decongestants, steroids and some medicines for high blood pressure, asthma or depression can cause sleeping difficulties as a side-effect. If you are taking any medication and aren't sleeping well discuss your medication with your doctor to see if it is causing the problem.

ELEVEN

Sleep Disorders

SLEEPING TOO MUCH?

You may find it a little odd to discuss the problem of sleeping too much here but if you are having problems getting to sleep at night you could well find yourself falling asleep during the day and sleeping in too long in the morning. Once the cause of your sleeping problems has been resolved, you should start to get a good night's sleep. However, if you are still falling asleep in the daytime even after a week or two of getting enough sleep at night, you should consult your GP to rule out the possibility of a sleep-related breathing disorder, of which the most common are sleep apnoea (opposite) and snoring (*see pages 107–111*).

NARCOLEPSY (DAYTIME SLEEPINESS)

This is an uncommon condition that has often not been recognised by doctors. There are two main symptoms: you feel sleepy in the daytime, with sudden uncontrollable attacks of sleepiness, even when you are with other people; and you suddenly lose control of your muscles and collapse when you are angry, laughing or excited – this is called cataplexy. You may also find that you:

- can't speak or move when falling asleep or waking up (sleep paralysis)
- hear odd sounds or see dream-like images (hallucinations)
- run on 'auto-pilot' – you have done things but can't remember doing them, as if you had been asleep
- wake with hot flushes during the night

The cause for this condition has recently been discovered – a lack of a substance called orexin or hypocretin. Treatment consists of taking regular exercise and having a night-time routine. Depending on the pattern of symptoms, medication may be helpful – an antidepressant or a drug that increases wakefulness, such as modafinil, which your GP can prescribe.

SLEEP APNOEA

Sleep apnoea is a term that means not breathing properly during sleep. It is the most common type of sleep-related breathing disorder. Although there are many different types of sleep apnoea, by far the most common is obstructive sleep apnoea (OSA). OSA involves a physical obstruction of the upper airways, as opposed to central sleep apnoeas which involve a failure in breathing control.

People who have sleep apnoea can stop breathing for 10–30 seconds at a time when they are sleeping, and this can occur several hundreds of times a night. Most at risk are middle-aged, overweight men who snore, have a collar size of over 16 and experience problems staying awake during the day in meetings or while watching television, driving or reading.

A person with sleep apnoea may wake up momentarily to resume breathing each time there is an airway obstruction. The unsuspecting person may think they have actually slept the whole night when in fact they have woken up to 500 times to resume breathing! Recent research suggests that sleep apnoea may cause heart disease, and that people with apnoea may be at risk of nocturnal sudden death.

> **George**, a 43-year-old executive, had a history of snoring with pauses in breathing and daytime sleepiness. For the past two years he had not slept with his wife because of his snoring and he had gained nearly two stone in weight. His wife described a pattern of loud snoring, cessation of breathing and a loud snort followed by the resumption of breathing. He woke up in the morning feeling exhausted and had to fight to stay awake during the day and at times during conversations. He also had difficulty keeping his eyes open as he drove to work, and fell asleep watching television and while reading. When George finally went to see his doctor he was immediately referred to a sleep specialist who diagnosed him as having severe sleep apnoea.

DEALING WITH SLEEP APNOEA

Talk to your GP if you think you have sleep apnoea. Some cases of sleep apnoea can be cured by weight loss and by sleeping on your side. The first stage of treatment for any kind of sleep apnoea is to look at lifestyle. Initial recommendations will include weight loss and cutting out alcohol and tobacco. Further treatment will depend on how severe the sleep apnoea is. In mild cases, drugs or medication may be prescribed; in moderate cases a continuous positive airway pressure device (CPAP) may be recommended. This is often considered the gold standard of sleep apnoea treatment because of its effectiveness and consists of an air pump and a mask that is worn over the nose and mouth at night. More serious cases of sleep apnoea are treated surgically.

Your GP may ask you to go to a sleep clinic for a sleep study. During your sleep study, you may try different levels of air pressure with a CPAP device to see which level helps. In general, heavier people and people who have severe apnoea need higher air pressures.

SNORING AND SLEEP APNOEA

Many sleep apnoeas are associated with snoring but not all snoring is a sign of apnoea. Between 30 to 40 per cent of adults snore and it is caused by vibrations of the tissues behind the mouth and nose when a person breathes in during sleep. If sleep apnoea is the case, the individual will snore and gasp very loudly. Primary snoring (snoring not due to apnoea) is not life-threatening and will not cause chronic fatigue during the day. It can, however, lead to sleeping problems for bed partners of snorers (*see pages 147–9*).

SLEEP TALKING

Sleep talking (somniloquy) happens in any stage of sleep. Most people associate sleep talking with REM sleep. REM or 'rapid eye movement' is the stage of sleep in which we have our most vivid and memorable dreams. However, the truth is that sleep talking tends to happen during the transition from one stage of sleep to another.

Sleep talking that happens at a light sleep level tends to be more understandable. Talking during deep sleep is more likely to be mutterings or gibberish. People who suffer from sleep apnoea are more prone to sleep talking as their breathing problems mean they don't always attain the deepest level of sleep.

Sleep talking can also be triggered by stressful situations or occur at times of poor health. Stress and illness cause poor sleep cycles. Other causes of sleep talking are a lack of proper sleep and eating the wrong foods near bedtime. To reduce sessions of sleep talking, eat healthily and take time to relax and de-stress each day. Make sure you are getting the proper amount of sleep you need each night.

SLEEPWALKING

Sleepwalking (somnambulism) can range from sitting up in bed while asleep to full-blown walking. Sleepwalkers do not appear to be asleep because their eyes are wide open with dilated pupils but they are deeply asleep. People who sleepwalk are not acting out their dreams but can do some pretty unusual things ranging from making themselves a meal to going on shopping sprees.

Sleepwalking can be triggered by illness, sleep deprivation and emotional upset, and episodes last from a few seconds to 30 minutes. Injuries and falls are common so keeping a safe environment is essential. It would also be wise to seek advice from your GP and perhaps be referred to a sleep clinic.

If you sleepwalk, you will appear (to other people) to wake from a deep sleep. You will then get up and do things. These may be quite complicated, like walking around or going up and down stairs. This can land you in embarrassing (and occasionally dangerous) situations. Unless someone else wakes you up, you will remember nothing about it the next day. A sleepwalker should be guided gently back to bed and should not be woken up, as sleepwalkers are hard to wake. It may be necessary to take precautions to protect them or others from injury. You may need to lock doors and windows, or lock away sharp objects, like knives and tools.

TWELVE

Food and Sleep

What does food have to do with a good night's sleep? Actually a great deal! Some foods and eating habits contribute to restful sleep while others keep you awake. It's as simple as that.

EATING BEFORE BEDTIME

*Every Friday night, **Luke**, 21, goes out with his colleagues for a pizza or a Chinese. He really enjoys the occasion but finds it impossible to get to sleep that night. At first he put it down to being excited about the approaching weekend, but one week when the meal out was cancelled and he had a light home-cooked meal instead, he slept like a log. Luke still goes out with his colleagues on Fridays but he has learned to be extremely careful about what he orders. If he overeats, especially cheese or monosodium glutamate (MSG), he pays for it with a terrible night's sleep.*

Nothing illustrates the effect food can have on our sleep more than the advice we've all heard about not eating a big meal before bedtime. However, many of us choose to ignore this advice. Sometimes we convince ourselves that a big meal will actually help us get to sleep by exhausting our body as it tries to digest it. It's tempting logic, but research evidence points in the opposite direction. A large meal asks our circulatory system to move more blood to our digestive tract. It asks our stomach to secrete more gastric acid. It asks our pancreas to become more active and produce digestive enzymes. It asks the smooth muscles around our intestines to become active. In short, a large meal does anything but relax us. Additionally, our digestive tracts are set up to work best when we are standing. Lying down results in gravity pulling the 'wrong way' to help food digest.

Sleep is the least physically demanding part of the day, and the least logical target for release of food energy and nutrients. We tell ourselves we've had a hard day and we're starved, but at this point we don't actually need the energy release any more. We need the nourishment before the hard day, and hopefully it will make the day less difficult.

At the opposite end of the scale there is the problem of going to bed hungry. This also interferes with sleep, usually by failing to keep the brain supplied with enough glucose (sugar) so it wakes you up when supplies are low. A small snack in the hour before bed is usually not problematic if you are truly hungry, but the ideal solution is to time your last meal two hours before bedtime.

As a rule it is best to eat a larger meal at lunchtime and a smaller meal in the evening. Your body needs to be resting, not digesting, at night.

WHAT NOT TO EAT AND DRINK BEFORE BED

ALCOHOL

Drinking alcohol at night is commonly believed to be helpful for a good night's sleep but this is a myth. Drinking can make you fall into a deep sleep but about three hours later, when the effects of the alcohol wear off, you will wake up exhausted and sleep will continue to be disrupted for the rest of the night.

Drinking also affects breathing so you are more likely to snore, and because it has a diuretic effect you are likely to need several visits to the toilet during the night. Over time, alcohol-induced sleep becomes increasingly less restful, so sleepiness will become a constant fact of life. This isn't to say you should give up alcohol but don't use it as a sleeping pill.

SAFE DRINKING

Women should drink no more than two to three units of alcohol per day and no more than 14 units of alcohol a week. Men should drink no more than three to four units of alcohol a day and no more than 21 units a week. One unit is considered to be 8 grammes of alcohol. Often units are quoted as being one small glass of wine, half a pint of beer or one pub measure of spirits.

CAFFEINE

You should avoid caffeinated drinks and foods – coffee, tea, many soft drinks and chocolate – several hours before bed. This is because caffeine is a stimulant that is known to cause problems with sleep. It's a natural chemical that activates the central nervous system, which means that it can make you feel more alert during the day and cause insomnia at night. It can also make some people feel jittery and slightly ill.

Caffeine enters the bloodstream very quickly and takes about 10–15 minutes to perk you up; it then stays in your system for three to eight hours afterwards. If you drink caffeinated drinks too close to bedtime, chances are it will keep you awake. What 'too close' means is totally individual, and sensitive people should stop drinking caffeine at least eight hours before bedtime (that means by 3pm if you go to bed around 11pm). You need to find what your caffeine cut-off time is during the day but don't experiment on a night when you absolutely must get a good night's sleep. Bear in mind, too, that even if you have no problems falling asleep after drinking caffeine, the quality of your sleep may be affected.

Most people expect to find caffeine in coffee, tea, cocoa and caffeinated cola drinks but it's important to know that it is also present in a lot of other places too, including chocolate, desserts and over-the-counter medications such as cold medicines and painkillers. Green tea has many wonderful health-boosting properties but you shouldn't drink it in the evening either as it does contain caffeine.

SMOKING

Aside from the damaging effects of smoking on your health, nicotine stimulates brain activity and increases blood pressure and heart rate. All these factors will stop you getting a good night's sleep. Studies show that when smokers quit, the quality of their sleep improves – yet another incentive to give up.

SUGAR

If your diet during the day is too high in refined sugar this will have a negative effect on your blood sugar levels and the quality of your sleep. Refined sugar is found in many foods such as:

➤ sweets
➤ pastries
➤ cakes
➤ fizzy drinks
➤ baked beans

➤ ketchup
➤ white bread, rice and pasta

Once digested, sugar shoots into your bloodstream, giving you an instant high but then departs from your system leaving you feeling drained and in need of another sweet fix. It's a vicious cycle that can go on and on. In the long term, these sugar highs and lows can cause hormonal imbalances, weight gain (the sugar your body doesn't use for energy gets turned into fat) and sleeping problems. To reduce this risk you need to cut down on the amount of sugar and refined foods in your diet and increase your intake of:

➤ whole foods and grains
➤ legumes
➤ nuts
➤ seeds
➤ fruits and vegetables

These foods release energy slowly into your system so you have balanced blood sugar levels and sustained energy without hunger pangs. You should also make sure you don't skip meals as going for long periods without eating will unsettle your blood sugar levels and cause potential sleeping problems. Aim to have a hearty breakfast followed by a mid-morning snack, such as some fruit and a handful of nuts and seeds, then a healthy lunch, a mid-afternoon snack and a light supper.

WHAT YOU SHOULD EAT FOR A GOOD NIGHT'S SLEEP

Foods that contain a substance called tryptophan promote sleep. Tryptophan is converted to an amino acid called L-tryptophan and produces a brain chemical called serotonin. This is essential for sleep and has been called the 'sleep hormone'.

A 2005 study of people with chronic insomnia found that diet made a big difference. After three weeks, those who ate foods with high amounts of tryptophan with carbohydrates, or who took pharmaceutical-grade tryptophan supplements, had improvements on all measures of sleep. Food sources worked just as well as the supplements.

Foods high in tryptophan include:

➤ almonds
➤ turkey
➤ bananas
➤ dairy products
➤ cabbage
➤ kidney beans
➤ oats
➤ spinach
➤ wheat
➤ poultry
➤ eggs
➤ tofu and soya products
➤ Marmite

For best results you need to eat foods that contain tryptophan with healthy carbohydrates. For example, combine turkey with a small baked potato; pasta with Parmesan cheese; tofu with stir-fry; tuna with salad and wholewheat bread. That's because in order for sleep-inducing tryptophan to work, it has to make its way to the brain. Carbohydrates cause the release of insulin, which helps tryptophan reach the brain and cause sleepiness. Without the carbohydrates the tryptophan is up against too many competing amino acids and can't reach the brain.

EATING AND SLEEPING

To find out if your sleeping problems are food related it might be helpful to keep an evening meal and sleep diary (*see pages 136–8*). However, if you don't think there is a connection between what you eat and how you sleep, remember that being healthy generally involves eating healthily, and healthy people tend to sleep better.

A healthy, whole-food diet rich in fruits, vegetables, whole grains, nuts, seeds, legumes and oily fish is the best diet for balancing your blood sugar levels and promoting a good night's sleep. You should also eat little and often and avoid going for more than three hours without food.

Making sure your diet is full of fresh whole foods will also help you avoid eating too much salt, additives and preservatives, which are often found in ready meals and processed and refined foods. A high intake of salt (sodium) is linked to an increased risk of high blood pressure. Not only can additives and preservatives – such as E numbers and monosodium glutamate (MSG) – trigger allergic reactions and cause head-aches, weight gain and poor concentration, they can also act as stimulants and stop you having a good night's sleep. Get used to reading labels so you can avoid them.

NUTRIENTS FOR HEALTHY SLEEP

If you're eating healthily you should be getting all the nutrients you need for healthy sleep. However, you may want to pay special attention to the following nutrients which have been shown to be natural relaxants and particularly important for healthy sleep:

➤ **B vitamins:** These are most closely linked to a good night's sleep and the control of tryptophan – especially vitamin B3 found in lean meat, oily fish, wheat germ and dried fruit; vitamin B6 found in whole grains, wheat germ, bananas and walnuts; and vitamin B12 found in dairy products, eggs and lean meat.

➤ **Iron:** Low levels of iron have been associated with restless legs syndrome, a cause of sleep disruption (*see pages 100–101*). Food sources include spinach, lean meat and poultry.

➤ **Magnesium and calcium:** Magnesium and calcium deficiency has been associated with wakefulness during the night. Sources of magnesium include bananas, wheat germ, nuts, seeds and whole grains, and sources of calcium include dairy products and green leafy vegetables.

➤ **Zinc:** Zinc promotes restful, restorative sleep. Sources include dairy products, oats and pumpkin seeds.

SUPPERS AND SNACKS FOR GOOD SLEEP

The best type of supper for blood sugar sustenance and a good night's sleep generally comprises:

➤ protein (such as lean meat, fish, eggs, tofu)
➤ vegetables
➤ a little carbohydrate (such as wholewheat bread, pasta and rice, as well as potatoes)
➤ a little healthy fat (such as olive oil, oily fish, nuts, seeds)

You could have, for example:

➤ scrambled eggs on wholegrain toast with some grated cheese
➤ chicken with stir-fried vegetables
➤ tuna in a baked potato with a crisp green salad
➤ pasta with Parmesan cheese
➤ turkey salad with a wholegrain roll and a scrape of butter

Stay away from foods that can cause indigestion, gas or heartburn. Pickles, garlic or fatty or spicy foods are best avoided at night. If you are sensitive to MSG you might induce insomnia by eating a late-night pizza or Chinese takeaway.

If you're going to eat before bed, opt for a small carbohydrate-based snack that includes some protein and fat. This could be:

➤ hummus and wholewheat bread
➤ a banana with a handful of seeds
➤ a small bowl of whole- or oat-grain cereal
➤ a biscuit with milk

You may also want to include a few of the snooze foods listed below in your supper and bedtime snack. Don't go overboard and eat too much at night, though. Heed the good sleep advice I give all my clients: 'Don't dine after nine.'

SNOOZE FOODS

➤ **Bananas:** They're practically a sleeping pill in a peel. In addition to a bit of soothing melatonin and serotonin, bananas contain magnesium, a muscle relaxant.

➤ **Chamomile tea:** Chamomile has a calming and soothing effect on the body and is a traditional sleep-inducing remedy. Having a mug of chamomile tea instead of tea or coffee after dinner helps to improve the quality and quantity of our slumber.

➤ **Warm milk:** It's not a myth. Milk contains some tryptophan – an amino acid that has a sedative effect – and calcium, which helps the brain use tryptophan. If you have a lactose intolerance there is evidence to suggest that non-milky herbal teas are just as effective in promoting a good night's sleep.

➤ **Lettuce:** This contains a substance called lactur carium that helps promote sleep by sedating the nervous system. A crisp green salad with supper is a good option for those who tend to have difficulty dropping off at night.

➤ **Honey:** Drizzle a little in your warm milk or herbal tea. Lots of sugar is stimulating, but a little glucose tells your brain to turn off orexin, a recently discovered neurotransmitter that's linked to alertness.

➤ **Potatoes:** A small baked potato can help clear away acids that can interfere with yawn-inducing tryptophan. To up the soothing effects, mash it with warm milk.

➤ **Oatmeal:** Oats are a rich source of sleep-inviting melatonin, and a small bowl of warm cereal with a splash of maple syrup or honey is comforting and filling.

➤ **Almonds:** A handful of these heart-healthy nuts can help you feel sleepy as they contain both tryptophan and a nice dose of muscle-relaxing magnesium.

➤ **Marmite:** A slice of toast with Marmite will release insulin, which helps tryptophan get to your brain where it's converted to serotonin and B vitamins to help you gently fall asleep.

➤ **Turkey:** It's the most famous source of tryptophan, but it works best when your stomach's basically empty, not overstuffed, and when there are some carbohydrates around. Put a lean slice or two on some wholewheat bread mid-evening, and you've got one of the best sleep-inducers in your kitchen.

CHANGE YOUR EATING HABITS FOR A BETTER NIGHT'S SLEEP

In a nutshell:

➤ Work out your caffeine cut-off time.
➤ Try to opt for nutrients that can help to facilitate sleep near bedtime.
➤ Experiment with snooze foods to work out which are best for you.
➤ Eat as healthily as you can during the day.
➤ Eat carefully for your evening meal: avoid heavy or greasy foods or foods that can trigger heartburn.
➤ If you need a snack before you go to bed, a glass of warm milk and a digestive or a turkey sandwich are fine.
➤ Eat at the table, not at your desk, in front of the television or in bed. Any of these will distract you from what and how much you are eating.
➤ Leave at least two hours between your last meal and bedtime.
➤ Give your meal a chance to digest and you'll get a better night's sleep.
➤ Pay attention to why you eat. If you eat when you are bored or stressed it is through habit; but if you want to assure a good night's sleep it's a habit you need to break.

THIRTEEN

Dealing with Insomnia

Still can't sleep? It's not that unusual. Nearly everybody has a hard time falling asleep now and again, and around 10 per cent of the general population is insomniac. Not only do they find it difficult to fall asleep, but they also wake several times during the night and feel fatigued the next day. When night time is a struggle you won't be getting the refreshing and restorative sleep you need, so before the situation gets out of hand and starts affecting your health I strongly advise you to find out what is keeping you awake.

KEEPING A SLEEP DIARY

To solve any problem, you have to identify it first. One reliable way to pinpoint your sleep problems is to keep track of each night's sleep (or lack of it). Used in the right way a sleep diary can be a helpful way to assess what or who may be preventing you from getting a good night's sleep. You need to use it for at least seven to 14 days to make it work for you.

GETTING STARTED

Take a large piece of blank paper and divide it into seven columns (for days of the week) and 19 rows. At the top of the first column, write the date on which you will start keeping your sleep diary, then put the next day's date in the next column and so on. Then label the rows with the following questions:

Morning questions:
Did you wake up by your alarm clock or naturally?
What time did you go to bed?
How long do you think it took to fall asleep?
How many times did you wake in the night and for what reason?
How long did you sleep in the night?
Did you sleep well?
Did your partner snore and/or wake you up?
What was your bedtime routine?

Evening questions:
How did you feel today?
Did you nap today?
Did you drink any tea or coffee today?
Did you have any alcohol today?
When was your evening meal?
What did you have for your evening meal and/or snack?
What is the temperature in your bedroom?
Did you take any medication?
Did you exercise today? If so, at what time, for how long and how vigorously?

After seven days, repeat the exercise with a new sheet of paper. After 14 days you will have a detailed picture of your sleep habits. Use the sleep diary to look for connections between good sleep days and bad sleep days. Pay particular attention to days when you reported feeling refreshed and awake in the morning. Do you see any connections between caffeine, alcohol or exercise? With all the facts in front of you, it will be easier for you to detect patterns that can help you self-diagnose your sleep problems.

Remember, something seemingly unimportant may hold the key to your problem so try to make a note of any changes to your daytime or sleeping routine. If you can't get to the bottom of the problem yourself, keep your sleep diary and show it to your doctor or a sleep specialist; they might see something you have missed.

WILL SLEEPING PILLS HELP?

People have used sleeping tablets for many years, but we now know that they are probably best used as a last resort and for short periods only. This is because they don't work for very long so you have to take more and more to get the same effect, and they can leave you tired and irritable the next day. In addition, some people become addicted to them. The longer you take sleeping tablets, the more likely you are to become physically or psychologically dependent on them.

If you have used or are using sleeping pills general advice is to use them only in emergencies or for short periods (less than two weeks). They may be helpful, for example, if you are under extreme stress or need to adjust quickly to shift work rotation. People who have been on sleeping tablets for a long time, are often advised to reduce the dose slowly after discussing it with their doctor.

Other medications that may disturb sleep are statins, fluoxetine, pseudoephedrine and steroids. (Bear in mind, however, that drug withdrawal can also cause sleep problems.) Talk to your GP if you are on any medication that may be interrupting your sleep.

Your GP may prescribe benzodiazepines, such as temazepam, for short-term sleep disturbances. However, they have side-effects and can impair the quality of your sleep. Antidepressants may also induce insomnia or excessive sleepiness.

OVER-THE-COUNTER SLEEP REMEDIES

You can buy several non-prescription sleep remedies at your chemist. These will often contain antihistamine, like you find in medicines for hay-fever, coughs and colds. They do work but they can make you sleepy well into the next morning so, again, I do not advise their use. If you do use them, take the warnings seriously and don't drive or operate heavy machinery the next day. Another problem is tolerance – as your body gets used to the substance, you need to take more and more to get the same effect. If you are taking any medication for your blood pressure (or any other sleeping tablets or tranquillisers), check with your doctor before using any over-the-counter remedy.

Herbal Sleep Remedies

Herbal alternatives are often based on a herb called valerian. Side-effects appear to be mild. Although there is a great deal of anecdotal evidence to suggest that it is effective, there still isn't enough scientific proof. One recent study declared that valerian was safe but not effective. It probably works best if you take it nightly for two to three weeks or more. It doesn't seem to work so well if you take it occasionally. As with the antihistamines, you need to be careful about the effects lasting into the following morning. If you are taking any medication for your blood pressure (or any other sleeping tablets or tran-quillisers), check with your doctor before using any herbal remedy.

MELATONIN SUPPLEMENTS

Melatonin is a hormone produced in the brain by the pineal gland, from the amino acid tryptophan (*see page 129*). The synthesis and release of melatonin are stimulated by darkness and suppressed by light, suggesting the involvement of melatonin in circadian rhythm and sleep and waking cycles. Levels of melatonin in the blood are highest prior to bedtime.

Studies show that low-level melatonin supplementation may help promote sleep in some poor sleepers if given during the day. Rather than affecting sleep itself, melatonin is thought to help reset your internal body clock so that your chances of getting a good night's sleep are improved. It doesn't seem to be addictive or to have any side-effects. Caution is advised, however, if you are considering taking melatonin supplements to aid sleep or jet lag. Despite its widespread use, little is actually known about the long-term safety of these supplements and more research needs to be done. It's a potent hormone, which suggests that melatonin should be taken *only* under medical supervision. It is also not readily available in the UK, so you would need to get a prescription from your GP.

* * *

For short-term insomnia, safe and responsible use of both pre-scribed and over-the-counter sleeping pills can be useful but it is always far better to follow the sleep strategies outlined in this book, and if that doesn't help to consult your doctor. If you use recreational drugs like marijuana to help you go to sleep it's also best to wean yourself off them, as although such drugs can have a sedative effect in the short term, long-term use is associated with an increased risk of insomnia.

DON'T TOSS AND TURN

If you can't sleep, don't lie there tossing and turning. Get up and do something you find relaxing. Read, listen to quiet music (without words, as these can be stimulating), do some light housework or re-make your bed (as if you are starting to get into bed again). After a while you should feel tired enough to go to bed again. The next morning, however hard it is, try to avoid the temptation of sleeping in as this will only make it harder for you to sleep the following night.

Don't beat yourself up if you do have a bad night or two; it's perfectly normal and won't do you any harm. Try not to worry; keep things in perspective. The more you worry about not sleeping, the less likely you are to sleep well. And the chances are if you sleep badly one night you'll sleep like a log the next, especially if you are doing regular exercise and following a bedtime routine.

STILL CAN'T SLEEP?

If you've read the advice in Chapters 3 to 12 and tried the tips in this chapter but you still can't sleep, go and see your doctor before self-medicating with over-the-counter sleeping pills. You can talk over any problems that may be stopping you from sleeping. Your doctor will make sure that your sleeplessness is not being caused by a physical illness, a prescribed medicine or emotional problems. If no physical cause is found for your sleeping problems, and depression is ruled out (a common symptom of depression is poor quality sleep), your doctor can recommend a cognitive therapist or a sleep therapist.

COGNITIVE BEHAVIOURAL THERAPY

There is some evidence that cognitive behavioural therapy (CBT) can be helpful if your sleeplessness has gone on for a long time. CBT involves talking with a therapist to address your beliefs, assumptions and attitudes (in this case, about sleep), all of which may be preventing you from getting the sleep you need.

Misconceptions regarding sleep can involve unrealistic expectations ('I must get eight hours of sleep every night'), exaggeration of the consequences of not getting enough sleep ('If I don't get a full eight hours of sleep tonight a catastrophe will happen'), faulty thinking about the cause of your insomnia ('My insomnia is completely caused by my anxiety about work'), and misconceptions about healthy sleep practices. CBT can help correct these misconceptions and replace them with positive sleep attitudes and behaviours that can help you get a healthy night's sleep. It is often used in conjunction with stim-ulus control (learning to associate the bedroom with rest and quality sleep), relaxation techniques and, in some cases, sleep restriction.

Here is a typical exercise a CBT therapist might suggest: Before going to bed, anticipate what you might worry about in bed and write it down. Another method is to sit with your eyes closed and imagine your worry as if it were a balloon floating in the air and mentally burst it to de-clutter your mind. A cogni-tive therapist would also encourage a person with sleeping problems to have a set worry time during the day, and if worry occurs at other times to tell themselves that they will worry only in their set worry time. The idea is to show the person that they are in control of their worry and not the other way around.

Insomniacs can develop extremely negative thoughts about themselves when they can't sleep. For example, 'I can't even fall asleep. I don't do anything right.' This negative thinking can make it even harder to fall asleep. CBT helps deal with this negative thinking head-on during the day, helping emotional response to be countered during the night.

WHEN TO VISIT A SLEEP SPECIALIST

If you've been having problems sleeping for two weeks or more, and nothing in this chapter seems to help, you should consult your doctor immediately. They can examine you and decide if you need to see a sleep specialist. If you are referred to a sleep specialist and perhaps diagnosed with a sleep disorder, try not to panic; sleep disorders are not rare. They can, however, have a serious effect on your health and wellbeing, so the sooner they are diagnosed and treated the better.

'For five years I suffered from insomnia. It affected all parts of my life: my career, my children and my relationship with my partner which broke down under the strain. My exhaustion left me too tired to talk and at my lowest point I was only sleeping for 30-minute bursts. Every aspect of my life suffered. It was as if my very being was sucked out of me. My eyes felt scratchy, my head fuzzy and my limbs heavy. Imagine having the worst jet lag 24/7. I had almost resigned myself to this hopeless situation when I saw a relaxation CD aimed at insomniacs. I sent off for one. What did I have to lose? On the eighth night of listening to the gentle music on the tape I had my first sound sleep in five years. It was a miracle. I had so much energy. I continued listening to the CD every night for several weeks and soon I was into a good sleep routine. I'm in bed by 11pm and wake by myself at 7am. Unless you've had insomnia you have no idea how much it tears your life apart. When I was suffering from it I felt like a zombie – now I feel alive, human, again.' JANE, 38

Many people simply aren't aware that they have a sleeping disorder and that it can be treated. It may take a while to find the right treatment or therapy if your insomnia is severe but it is vital that you seek medical help. I've seen how insomnia can damage health and wellbeing if left untreated, and how more often than not, simple lifestyle changes, stress management and, if needed, medication can make a person feel alive again.

FOURTEEN

Sleeping Together

If you spend sleepless nights listening to your partner's loud snores, or regularly wake freezing because your partner has won the duvet war, or frequently can't get comfortable because they want a firm mattress and you prefer something softer, take comfort in the fact that you're not alone.

SLEEPING APART, TOGETHER

In my work as a physiotherapist I visit many patients in their homes and see a multitude of different sleeping arrangements. I have noticed time and time again that an increasing number of couples prefer to sleep in separate rooms, or find that their sleeping problems are resolved when they decide to sleep separately. More often than not this has nothing to do with their relationship or with problems in their sex life, and everything to do with their urgent need for a better night's sleep. Often this starts when one partner has an episode of illness, such as a cough, heavy cold or back pain, and moves temporarily to another room (or to the sofa) so as not to disturb their partner, and they both enjoy such a good night's sleep that they decide to keep it that way.

> **Mike**, 41, had recently been diagnosed with sleep apnoea and was given a CPAP (continuous passive airways pressure) device to help keep his airways open. This took a

*while for him to get used to and his snoring was still a problem. In the meantime, his wife **Lauren** started work full-time and urgently needed a good night's sleep. They made a pact: Sunday to Wednesday they would sleep in separate bedrooms and Thursday to Saturday together, with Lauren wearing her ear-plugs.*

Research by the UK Sleep Council found one in four of us regularly retreats to a spare room or sofa for a restful and refreshing night's sleep. In a 2007 survey by the National Association of Home Builders, builders and architects predicted that more than 60 per cent of custom-built houses would have dual master bedrooms by 2015.

SLEEPING APART

If you do prefer to sleep alone, this isn't a sign that your relationship is in trouble; quite the opposite in fact.

It's often assumed that as soon as you move in with someone, start a new relationship or get married you are automatically going to sleep together. However, if your partner has irritating sleeping habits or likes to keep different hours from you – for example, if you are a lark and they are an owl – this can cause a lot of tension in a relationship.

It's also worth pointing out that men and women sleep differently. Men have more awakenings than women but women report worse sleep, perhaps because hormonal fluctuations due to the menstrual cycle can disrupt sleep; not to mention the fact that women with curves have different mattress needs to men without curves. In short, men and women have different sleep needs.

Statistics show that people who sleep poorly have a higher divorce rate – so if you persist in sharing a bed despite having your sleep disrupted, you risk not just poor performance at work, reduced concentration and poor health but problems in your relationship too. So don't ignore sleep problems in your relationship.

If your partner is keeping you awake at night because of snoring or incompatible sleeping habits, and this is causing you to feel anger and resentment during the night and to feel irritable, tired and moody during the day, the sensible advice is to sleep in separate rooms.

If this isn't possible, either because you haven't got a spare room or because you or your partner really don't want to sleep alone, the following tips will help you deal with typical problems that can make sleeping with your partner difficult.

SNORING PARTNER

(See also Chapter 10.)

*The only way **Sally** can get off to sleep when **Steve** is around is with the window open to drown out his snoring with the noise of traffic. Somehow it is easier to fall asleep with the continuous noise of the passing traffic than with Steve's on-off snoring. Even though she adores Steve, Sally is quite happy to spend three nights of the week in bed alone to catch up on her four nights of traffic noise.*

Fifteen million British adults live with a snoring partner, depriving them of an average of two hours' sleep a night, according to a study by the British Snoring and Sleep Apnoea Association (BSSAA). Snoring and sleep apnoea – where someone stops breathing for about 30 seconds before starting again – are the biggest problems seen by sleep clinics, and can wreck relationships.

WHAT YOU CAN DO

One thing you might want to do if your partner snores is to record them snoring. A normal tape recorder or video camera will do. Often the first step in coping with snoring is getting the snorer to believe there is a problem. With the evidence in your hands, you can move on to fixing the problem.

Next you should encourage your partner to find the cause of their snoring (*try the tests on pages 110–11 and at www.britishsnoring.co.uk*). Snoring can be down to breathing through the mouth, so an adhesive chin strip can help keep the mouth closed; or, if it's the result of a stuffy nose, a nasal spray could help. If your partner stops breathing at intervals during the night, this indicates sleep apnoea, which can be linked to conditions including high blood pressure and diabetes, so encourage them to see their GP, who can refer them to a sleep clinic.

You could also try nudging your partner to wake them up, give them a shove or say 'Tut, tut'. If they are just as sleep-deprived as you, it'll motivate them to seek help for the problem.

Another strategy is to go to bed first. If you are in deeper stages of sleep when your partner comes to bed, their snoring is less likely to interrupt your sleep.

Ear-plugs can be useful (*see pages 63–64*). It may take a little time getting used to sleeping with something in your ears, but it's worth the effort to be able to get a restful night's sleep. Make sure that your snorer knows to wake you up when the alarm goes off.

You may also want to consider buying a white noise machine. These are programmed with continuous sounds that make noises like snoring or creaky floorboards less intrusive while you sleep.

Ben and Bella had been together for just three years. Ben, a smoker, had always had chronic sinusitis and snored. Bella also snored. They settled on a plan of action. Whoever got off to sleep first stayed in their bed and the other partner would sleep in the spare room. They agree that their arrangement isn't ideal but at least they both sleep.

RESTLESS NIGHTS

Steve kicks and lashes out uncontrollably when he sleeps. After several weeks of enduring bruises, Michelle finally decided that it was safer for her to sleep in a separate room.

If your partner tosses and turns during the night, or even kicks you, this can make it extremely hard not just to sleep but to sleep safely. You can also be woken if your partner has an allergy which causes scratching, or if your partner simply moves a lot in their sleep.

WHAT TO DO

Your partner could have restless legs syndrome (*see pages 100–101*) or a related condition called periodic limb movement during sleep, so a checkup by their GP is advised to rule this out.

If allergies are the problem, antihistamines can be the answer; or simply cleaning your bedroom and airing your bed more during the day may help. Check, too, that you aren't using washing powders that are causing irritations.

Buying a bigger bed makes sense. Many standard double beds are simply too small so buy the biggest bed you can. If this isn't possible, try a mattress that zips down the middle or put two single mattresses on one bed; this way you are far less likely to be woken with a kick.

BODY HEAT

David has always liked to wrap himself up and sleep in a cocoon of sheets and duvet. This was fine until his partner, Jenny, moved in. Night time became a battle for the duvet; a battle that finally ended when Jenny went out and bought two single duvets.

One of the most common reasons people find it hard to share a bed is different temperature preferences, which can lead to fights over the duvet.

WHAT TO DO

The obvious solution is to buy and use separate single duvets. You can then both choose the duvet weight and comfort level that you want. Don't forget, too, that a cool room is optimal for good sleep. Wearing lightweight natural fibres such as cotton in bed will also help regulate body heat.

LARKS VERSUS OWLS

Being in a relationship with someone who keeps different hours can be challenging.

Shannon, 55, has always been an early riser, and typically likes to be in bed by 10.30pm. Jon, 56, is more nocturnal and never gets into bed before 1am. They settled their differences by turning their spare room into another bed-room and regularly sleep apart.

You like to be tucked up by 10.30pm, but your partner clambers in after midnight and reads, waking you for a chat or a cuddle. The next morning your alarm goes off at 6.30 and your partner is grumpy because they've been woken up and they wanted to sleep in till at least 7.30.

WHAT TO DO

If you don't want to sleep separately, replace any bedside lamps with reading lights as they are less disruptive. You should also both invest in an eye mask to block out all light. If you're a lark and your partner is an owl, it's probably best if only your partner wears ear-plugs. This is because one of you needs to be able to hear an alarm, and it's easier for a lark to sleep through when an owl goes to bed than it is for an owl to sleep through when a lark gets up. We sleep more lightly in the second half of the night, so if one of you gets up early, the other is likely to wake more easily.

Larks who sleep with owls should also try to put their clothes out ready in another room so that they don't rustle around in the morning when they are getting dressed. Owls should return the favour at night by getting ready for bed in another room. Pay attention also to the layout of your bed-room and plan it so that an owl does not have to pass the lark's side of the bed at night.

CATS AND DOGS

Unless you can't bear to be without your pet during the night, cats and dogs in the bedroom aren't really a good way to improve your chances of a good night's sleep. Their movements and noises during the night can prove to be a big problem. You might want to think about getting them to sleep in the kitchen or in a kennel instead so that you get a good night's sleep and have the energy to play with them during the day.

SLEEP POSITIONS FOR COUPLES

When you sleep together, some sleep experts recommend 'spooning'. This is the position where people sleep nested together like spoons. This is believed to increase intimacy and lower stress but may also worsen back pain and snoring.

Sometimes people worry because their spouse is sleeping with their back to them or seems to be far away in the bed. Don't jump to conclusions; there is no 'good' or 'bad' sleep position in a relationship.

BEST SOLUTION: COMPROMISE

So what do you do if you have different sleep preferences? Find ways to compromise by following the guidelines above. If that doesn't work, be realistic and consider separate bedrooms or twin beds.

Although some couples worry that sleeping in twin beds or having separate rooms will hurt their intimacy with one another, many sleep experts believe that sleeping apart when there are sleep issues can save a relationship and actually increase intimacy. If you believe in your relationship, trust each other, and communicate well with one another about the issue of lack of sleep in your lives, sleeping apart won't hurt your intimacy. Asking the question, 'Your room or mine?' can increase your sexual delight with your spouse.

When couples first start seeing each other and sleeping together, they are willing to sacrifice comfort to be close to their partner. After a while, when emotional closeness is assured, many people just want to have a good night's sleep again. This isn't selfish, distant or unromantic – it's just practical.

FIFTEEN

Travelling and Overtime

JET LAG

Whether we travel for work or pleasure, many of us have experienced the mental and physical upset we call jet lag. This occurs when the body clock is disrupted by crossing a number of time zones. To make matters worse, not all internal body functions adjust at the same rate. So your sleep-wake cycle may adjust more quickly than your temperature, while your digestion may be on yet another schedule.

Symptoms of jet lag can include fatigue, disorientation and an inability to sleep. This can cause business travellers to be less productive in meetings and less dynamic in presentations, tourists to be too tired to fully enjoy their holiday, and athletes and performers to be less on the ball, physically and mentally.

We are already one step ahead with our knowledge and understanding of the effects of jet lag, and this can help us reduce some of the frustrations we might feel from this change in our schedules. Use the tips in this chapter to help you work with your systems in an appropriate way.

Sam, *a 39-year-old management consultant heading up a division of a global firm, frequently flew out of London to Los Angeles. On his way home he would stop off in New York for meetings then catch a 'red eye' home so that he could be back at his desk the following morning. Sam represents thousands of businesspeople who are required to travel extensively to develop and maintain a presence in our global economy. Although Sam cut out junk foods and stimulants, he had to forgo regular exercise because with all the frequent flying he did there was no time. Last month he was on a plane, exhausted as usual, and experienced an episode of acute chest pain. Worried that he may have had a heart attack, he checked into hospital but doctors could find nothing wrong with him apart from sheer exhaustion. Sam had just experienced a panic attack.*

POTENTIAL SYMPTOMS OF JET LAG

DAYTIME DROWSINESS

Up to 90 per cent of travellers report fatigue and sleepiness during the day. However, if they give in and sleep during the day they may also have problems sleeping at night, making insomnia the next most common symptom of jet lag.

INSOMNIA

Travellers may find themselves unable to get to sleep at their normal bedtime. They may feel tired too early or wide-awake when it comes to their usual time to turn in. Insomnia in travellers is influenced primarily by the direction in which they travel (*see page 159*).

DECREASED ABILITY TO CONCENTRATE

Approximately two-thirds of travellers report poor concentration. They may find it hard to focus, think clearly and write or speak coherently.

DISORIENTATION

A large number of travellers also experience disorientation; they can't remember where they are, especially when they wake in the middle of the night.

SLOWER REACTION TIMES

Many travellers experience slower reaction times. This is especially dangerous if they need to cope with unfamiliar driving conditions in a new environment.

DIGESTIVE UPSETS

Up to half of travellers experience stomach upsets when they arrive at their destination. Their appetite may be poor or they may feel ravenous at strange times. Constipation is common, as is heartburn from eating foods at unusual times.

OTHER SYMPTOMS

➤ headaches
➤ irritability
➤ urinary problems
➤ menstrual cycle disturbances
➤ lowered immunity
➤ depression

CLOCKS FORWARD OR BACK

Even if you don't travel across time zones you may still experience mild symptoms of jet lag twice a year when the clocks go forward by one hour in March or back in October. Studies suggest that it takes people several days to fully readjust their sleep schedule after the time change. Fortunately, there are several ways to make the transition a little less tiring, including preparing for the change gradually.

Researchers report that adapting to the spring time change is more difficult than facing the end of Daylight Saving Time in October, which lengthens the day rather than shortens it. Every year the movement against Daylight Saving Time gathers momentum. Opponents claim that putting the clocks forward in March increases the risks of accidents on the roads, but at present there are no signs that the situation will change.

The following tips can help you beat fatigue and sleepless nights when the clocks change:

➤ Begin to rejig your sleeping routine a few days before the time change by hitting the sack earlier for a March clock change and later for an October change. You could start by going to bed 15 minutes earlier or later and then the next night 30 minutes, and so on.
➤ Get at least 15 minutes' exposure to sunlight, without sunglasses on, first thing in the morning.

The bright sunlight (or any bright light) tells your body's natural biological clock that it's time to wake up, and that same clock will then be set to tell your body it's time to go to sleep about 14–16 hours later.

➤ Reorganise your mealtime schedule by eating dinner earlier or later.

➤ Be careful when operating machinery or driving on the day of the time change.

➤ Avoid turning to caffeine to wake you up in the morning or alcohol at night to help you sleep. Eat properly, drink lots of water and remain physically active.

➤ Don't nap after 3pm.

HOW ALERT ARE YOU?

Pay attention to the signs of jet lag, such as bad mood, attention lapses and apathy, as they can negatively affect your health and work performance. If you recognise any jet lag symptoms the following tips may help:

➤ Stop what you are doing and, if possible, take a nap for an hour or 20 minutes.

➤ Go for a walk and do some gentle stretching exercises.

➤ Engage in social interaction (talk to someone).

➤ Turning on a bright light or listening to upbeat music can also help but only in the short term.

➤ Don't increase your caffeine intake during the day to perk you up, and don't rely on alcohol to help you drift off to sleep. Both these activities can result in lighter, more disrupted sleep.

➤ Prescription and non-prescription medications, including the use of melatonin supplements, are also not advised (*see pages 139–40*).

FACTORS THAT CONTRIBUTE TO JET LEG

The more time zones you travel across, the more noticeable your jet lag will be. The direction of your flight also matters greatly. When flying west – such as from London to New York – you are extending your day and going in the natural direction of your biological clock. This is because our internal body clock prefers to run for longer than 24 hours. In NASA studies of long-haul pilots, westward travel was associated with significantly better sleep quantity and quality than eastward trips. Flying eastwards – such as from New York to London – shrinks your day, in direct opposition to your internal clock's natural tendency. And because north-south and south-north flights do not involve time zone changes, you will not experience jet lag, although you may experience travel fatigue.

Night owls typically fare better than morning larks when flying westwards, but early risers tend to cope better when flying east. Your age and your personality will also affect your chances of experiencing the unpleasant symptoms of jet lag. It seems that the older you are the more likely you are to suffer, and in general easy-going, calm types with a flexible schedule tend to suffer less than more anxious types with a more regimented lifestyle. If you exercise regularly and are in good health and getting enough sleep, symptoms are also less severe.

STAYING ON HOME TIME

Because it can take the body clock anything from several days to several weeks to fully adjust to a new time zone, it may be less disruptive to keep yourself on your home time schedule if you are going to be away from home for only a short time (about 48 hours or less).

You need to do a bit of advance planning, but these steps will help:

➤ Calculate the time difference between your home time and the time at your destination.

➤ Consider when you would normally be asleep and awake on your home time compared to the times at the new destination.

➤ Make a note of the destination times that correspond with times when your body clock would be at maximum sleepiness at home (3–5am and, on a lesser level, 3–5pm).

➤ Try to avoid important business meetings scheduled at these times of maximum sleepiness at home.

➤ If you would normally be in darkness at home but it is light at your destination, try wearing sunglasses when you go out.

➤ When planning meals, try to keep your stomach on home time. So if it is dinner time at your destination but breakfast on your home time, try to have something light, rather than a full heavy dinner that your stomach may not be ready to digest.

IN FOR THE LONG HAUL

If your trip is going to be longer than 48 hours, you should start to adjust to your new time zone as soon as you board the plane and, if possible, three to five days before.

EASTBOUND TRAVEL TIPS

➤ Plan on going to bed and waking up earlier three to five days before you leave.

➤ After waking up, expose yourself to sunlight to help advance your biological clock. Remember, daylight is a powerful stimulant for your biological clock, and staying indoors can make jet lag worse.

➤ For the businessperson, try to schedule business meetings at your destination later in the afternoon instead of early in the morning, as you will probably be more alert later in the day.

➤ A day or two before or when leaving, set your watch to the destination's time so that you can start to psychologically adjust and anticipate the change.

➤ Eating your meals at 'destination times' before you leave can help you adjust.

➤ When you arrive don't be tempted to take a nap on your first day. It's much better to push yourself through the first day and then fall asleep early that evening when you are exhausted. If you need to stay awake, a brisk walk and plenty of exposure to sunlight will help keep your eyes open.

WESTBOUND TRAVEL TIPS

➤ If possible, plan on staying up later and getting up later three to five days before you leave.

➤ Take a long nap while on the plane if you can. This can shift your sleep cycles forward, and when you arrive you might not be as tired.

➤ If you arrive and the sun is still up, go ahead and expose yourself to the sunlight, as this can help delay the onset of sleep. Remember, it is much easier to adjust to westbound change because of the circadian rhythm's tendency towards a longer day.

➤ Sleep later in the morning if you can, and then expose yourself to sunlight after getting up.

➤ Eat at your destination's regular times. Remember, you can also do this before you arrive at your destination.

HOW TO SLEEP ON A PLANE

Sleeping through the night or even taking a power nap on a plane can be difficult. But with the proper preparations, a satisfactory snooze is possible for almost everyone.

➤ Reserve your seat in advance. Window seats give you a wall to lean on, and your neighbour won't need to disturb you on the way to the lavatory. Avoid completely the last row in the plane as the seats can't push back, and any seats just in front of the exit row as these tend to be noisy and busy. Think twice about bulkhead or aisle seats and any seat near the toilet. The nearer you are to the front of the plane, the quieter it is also likely to be.

➤ Buy and pack in your hand luggage the following: travel pillow and eye mask, ear-plugs, comfortable clothing, slippers and bottled water.

➤ Make sure that your body will be tired for the flight: before your departure, avoid sleeping in, napping or consuming caffeine, and try to get some exercise.

➤ Grab a pillow and blanket as soon as you get on the plane. Remember, your seat is reserved but blankets are not.

➤ Adjust your seat for maximum comfort. If you can't push it back far enough, try putting a pillow or blanket behind your lower back to make you more reclined.

➤ Ask what time the in-flight meal will be served. Falling asleep is easier on a full stomach. Eat a light meal or snack and avoid alcohol and spicy food – it will keep you awake. Make sure you drink plenty of water to stay hydrated.

➤ Warn your neighbours and flight attendant that you plan to fall asleep – they are less likely to disturb you – and put your seat belt on before drifting off, making sure it is clearly visible so that you won't be woken up by a flight attendant when the seat belt sign goes on.

➤ Set an alarm clock to wake you 40 minutes before you land so you have time to use the toilet, stretch and fully wake up.

DURING YOUR FLIGHT

As soon as you sit down, make sure you change your watch to the time of your destination and begin eating, living and, if necessary, sleeping by that time. You should also stay hydrated by drinking plenty of non-alcoholic, non-caffeinated fluids. Don't be afraid to ask your flight attendant for extra water. Dehydration can interfere with the process of resetting your body clock. Alcohol isn't advised as cabin pressure can raise your blood alcohol level, exacerbate the dehydration problem and interfere with the quality of your sleep. You should also avoid spicy foods and try not to overeat.

Get up out of your seat at regular intervals to walk and stretch. You can also do exercises like toe raises, isometric exercises (involving the static contraction of a muscle without any visible movement in the angle of the joint), stomach crunches and shoulder shrugs right in your seat. This keeps your blood flowing and prevents it from pooling at your extremities, a common phenomenon in pressurised cabins which can lead to deep vein thrombosis (DVT).

Other Tips

➤ Get up to wash your face, brush your teeth or just stand up for several minutes.

➤ Wear loose-fitting clothing that breathes.

➤ Avoid any snug footwear or high heels as it is quite possible that your feet will swell in transit, making your post-flight trek to baggage claim a nightmare.

➤ If you are going to do some work on the flight do it at the beginning of the journey and then sleep.

AFTER YOUR FLIGHT

Whether you are heading east or west, getting some exercise when you arrive – even a brisk walk – is a great idea. It will reduce stiffness and pain and help boost your mood and appetite.

Business executives, government officials, athletes and performers should delay business, performance or sporting trials until the second day abroad after a five-hour time shift. If they don't, mistakes are more likely to be made, negotiations will suffer, reputations will be tarnished and games lost.

(*For advice on ensuring a good night's sleep when staying away from home, see page 67.*)

DROWSY DRIVING

Sleepiness is second only to drunkenness as a cause of motorway accidents. Driving is one of the biggest threats to the safety of people with sleeping problems, particularly in monotonous situations such as motorway driving where lack of concentration and alertness can have fatal consequences. Therefore, making sure you are rested before beginning a drive is essential, and it is also important to know what to do when you start to feel tired when driving.

You may not feel sleepy when you get in your car and start your journey but if you are sleep-deprived the urge to sleep can become uncontrollable. Many drivers think they know when they have reached the point where they need to stop but research shows otherwise, indicating that many drivers fall asleep without realising it until it's too late.

Shift workers, the elderly and teenagers partying too hard are most at risk of drowsy driving. Studies also show that alcohol is involved in one-third of all accidents when the driver fell asleep. Sleep disorders, such as sleep apnoea (*see pages 119–21*), can also be a huge factor in causing road accidents, as can long working hours. One study revealed that 50 per cent of people who worked more than 50 hours a week had fallen asleep at the wheel. Other factors that contribute to increased risk of traffic accidents include unhealthy eating habits, late-night driving, driving alone and monotonous roads like motorways.

In terms of your biological clock, the times to be most vigilant when driving are 4–6am and 4–6pm, as these times are associated with the most road accidents.

WARNING SIGNS

If you find yourself experiencing any of the following you could be in danger of falling asleep at the wheel so pull off the road at the earliest opportunity, park in a safe place and take a 20-minute nap followed by a brief brisk walk. Most important of all, do not start driving again until you feel refreshed.

➤ Your eyelids feel heavy.
➤ You start feeling drowsy.
➤ Your eyes burn or feel strained; they close or go out of focus.
➤ Your vision is blurred.
➤ Your thoughts become disconnected.
➤ You have trouble keeping your head up.
➤ You keep yawning.
➤ You don't remember the last few miles you drove.
➤ You miss traffic signals and turnings.
➤ You keep jerking your car between lanes.
➤ You have problems maintaining the speed that you want.
➤ You drift off the road and narrowly miss crashing.

TEN TOP TIPS FOR PLANNING A LONG DRIVE

1. Start your drive feeling refreshed and rested.
2. Avoid driving after a full day of work and activities.
3. Plan your journey to include plenty of regular rest breaks with at least 15 minutes every two hours. Include an overnight stop if necessary.

4. Don't drive if taking medication that states you should not drive or operate machinery.
5. Avoid driving between midnight and 6am and be extra careful between 4pm and 6pm.
6. If you start to feel tired, stop where it is safe, have a non-alcoholic drink and take a short nap.
7. Adjust the car temperature so that it is not too warm.
8. Don't use cruise control.
9. Don't consume any alcohol before driving as just one drink can impair your ability to drive safely.
10. If you feel you need caffeine to stay awake you may be too tired to drive; postpone your journey and have a good night's sleep.

OVERTIME

As we move towards globalisation and a 24/7 work culture, there is increasing pressure on people to do overtime to increase income, status or simply to get a job done. Estimates suggest that 20 per cent of the workforce of industrialised countries have to work at unusual times. Many executives stay up late to take calls from other countries, and then there are those who are required to work shifts. Not surprisingly, the majority of shift workers are in a state of continuous jet lag, without ever leaving the country. Difficulty sleeping well because of the disruption to their circadian rhythm is so common that the International Classification of Sleep Disorders now recognises Shift Work Disorder or, as some like to call it, shift lag.

International research indicates that falling asleep on the job amongst shift workers is a common occurrence. In confidential surveys conducted, 80 per cent of shift workers interviewed admitted to 'nodding off' during the night shift.

Further studies found that night shift workers are twice as likely to make mistakes as their day shift colleagues. Not only do shift workers face a higher risk of injury during their working hours, they are also involved in more domestic (off-the-job) accidents than their day-working colleagues, and have more sick days and health problems than day workers. Shift lag is said to cost the UK £115–240 million per year in terms of work and road accidents alone. Aware of the problem, some companies will even pay for cabs home from work if you leave after a certain time.

It has been established that extreme fatigue is as harmful to worker performance as drunkenness. However, bear in mind that occasionally having to do overtime under pressure is not going to dull your performance; in fact it may even enhance it. If you can choose either to keep working late into the night or to leave work and come in earlier the following day, do what you are best suited for. Some people perform better first thing – they are the 'petrol engines' – while others take a while to get going and are more like 'diesel engines'. You need to find what works best for you.

CAN THE HUMAN BODY ADJUST TO UNUSUAL HOURS?

All living things (people, animals, even plants) have a circadian – or about 24-hour – rhythm. This affects when we feel sleepy and alert. Light and dark cycles set these circadian rhythms. For those who work unusual hours, however, the light and dark cycle doesn't change. Therefore, contrary to popular belief, a shift worker's circadian rhythm never adjusts; and whether you work the night shift or not, you are most likely to feel sleepy between midnight and 6am. And no matter how many years you work a night shift, sleeping during the day remains difficult.

SLEEP TIPS FOR SHIFT WORKERS

Although you can never fully adjust to shift work, or working at unusual hours, there are a number of strategies you can use to improve your sleep and stay alert. All the good night's sleep advice in this book still applies but the following tips are specifically designed to help you.

Before Work

➤ If you work evenings or nights, exposure to a sunlight box before going on shift can help reset your body clock.

➤ Take a nap two hours before your shift to help make up for sleep loss.

➤ If you work rotating shifts, ask your manager to schedule your shifts clockwise – day to evening to night. This means that your new shift will have a start time that is later than your last shift. Research from Harvard Medical School has shown that clockwise shifts result in increased productivity and work performance.

During Work

➤ Take a nap during a break in your shift. Even a nap of just 20–30 minutes can improve your alertness on the job.

➤ During night-time and evening shifts, expose yourself to full-spectrum bright light to help reset your body clock.

➤ Arrange for someone to pick you up after a night shift, or take a bus or cab home. Drowsy driving can put your life and the lives of other drivers at risk.

➤ Avoid caffeine during the last half hour of your shift because it will stop you falling asleep later.

➤ Go for a short wake-up walk at around 4am when your biological temperature is at its lowest.

➤ If you have a morning drive home after a night shift, wear dark glasses so the daylight doesn't reset your biological clock and your sleep cycle.

After Work

➤ Plan ahead for a major change in a shift-work schedule and begin to alter your sleep time a few days in advance. This will make it easier for your body to adjust.

➤ Avoid exposure to sunlight if you need to sleep during the day.

➤ Avoid alcohol after work if you need to sleep during the day as it can cause disrupted sleep.

➤ Make sure others in your home are aware of your work schedule. They should keep the home quiet when they know that you need to sleep.

➤ Try to relax, unwind and go through a regular bedtime routine before sleeping.

➤ Avoid heavy meals and strenuous exercise two hours before sleeping.

➤ Keep your bedroom cool and pitch dark. It might be a good idea to invest in some extra-thick curtains, an eye mask or other means of blocking out light.

➤ Maintain a consistent sleep schedule and make a good night's sleep a priority. Ask friends and family to avoid phone calls and visits during regularly scheduled sleep hours.

➤ Eat healthily and stay as physically fit as you can as this will increase your alertness on the job. Shift workers often turn to stimulants such as coffee or cigarettes to keep them awake and sedatives such as alcohol or sleeping pills to help them sleep. However, such aids have only short-term effects on alertness as tolerance soon develops. Persistent use may also increase the risk of dependence.

SURVIVING THE NIGHT: HOW EMPLOYERS CAN HELP

Employers can improve productivity and help increase job satisfaction by taking the following practical steps:

➤ Permit exercise. Several lab studies have shown that exercise during the night hours boosts alertness so permit the use of a stationary bike, a treadmill and free weights.

➤ Make sure there is always someone on duty for shift workers to consult with.

➤ Make sure healthy food options are available because the foods that tend to be available during the night hours – such as doughnuts and cheeseburgers – are hardest to digest at this time.

➤ Subsidise extended childcare and set tolerant policies when it comes to family emergencies.

➤ Allow napping on breaks. Several studies have shown that naps of 15–20 minutes provide an alertness boost that lasts several hours.

SIXTEEN

Sweet Dreams!

If you pay little attention to your dreams, you could be making a big mistake. Research shows that the images that flash through your head during the night are important for a good night's sleep and for your emotional wellbeing. And if you are one of those people who say they never dream, you're wrong. Everybody dreams – you just need to learn how to remember them.

THE LANGUAGE OF DREAMS

Groundbreaking new research on the dreaming mind reveals that dreams affect our lives far more than we may realise. Dreams, it is thought, are a way for our subconscious mind to communicate with our conscious mind. For example, if you dream of something that you fear – like going bankrupt or losing a loved one – it is your mind's way of helping you prepare for the worst if it happens. And if you dream of winning a race or being awarded a prize, this is your mind's way of boosting your confidence. Cognitive neuroscientists have also discovered that the rapid eye movement (REM) that occurs during the dream phase of sleep is linked to your ability to retain and recall new information.

Increasingly, psychologists are regarding dreams as a mood-regulating system that can help people work through problems, fears and challenges. While you sleep, your dreaming mind works a bit like an in-house therapist, comparing new situations with old memories. This is so that when you wake up, your conscious mind can work out what an old situation can teach you about your current situation.

The emotions you experience in your dreams can also help you deal with situations or challenges you are currently facing. For example, if you have recently had a traumatic experience like a relationship breakdown or losing a job, research shows that those whose dreams are more angry or emotional have the best chance of coping. Those whose dreams are bland or forgettable have less success working through their emotions and formulating a strategy to move forwards. In short, those with vivid and expressive dreams can literally dream their troubles away.

So it seems that REM sleep, the stage of sleep when you dream, is crucial for a truly good night's sleep.

REM SLEEP

REM sleep is characterised by tiny twitches of facial muscles and slight movements of the hands. Blood pressure rises; breathing and heart beat become faster; eyes dart rapidly around under closed eyelids as if looking at a moving object; and if you are a man you may have an erection. Researchers have discovered that when a sleeper is woken during REM sleep they typically say they have been dreaming.

Your brain is fully active during REM sleep, and during a typical night you will go through several REM phases lasting between 10 and 45 minutes. You are most likely to remember dreams that occur in the final stages of REM sleep, but you actually dream in every REM stage. Studies have shown that subjects repeatedly woken during REM sleep become anxious, bad tempered and irritable. This suggests that REM sleep and dreaming are essential for our emotional wellbeing. Therefore, although we still aren't sure why we need to sleep, it's possible to conclude that one of the reasons is that it enables us to dream.

NIGHT TERRORS

If you wake up terrified and screaming in the middle of the night you could have experienced a night terror. It is not a dream or nightmare but rather like having a panic attack in your sleep. People experiencing night terrors often don't know what made them feel so frightened, and often don't remember the episode in the morning.

Although commonly associated with childhood, night terrors are experienced by about one in 20 adults. Night terrors can occur on their own, without leading to sleepwalking. Like a sleepwalker, however, a person with night terrors will appear to wake suddenly from a deep sleep. They look half-awake and very frightened, but will usually settle back down to sleep without waking up completely. All you can do to help is sit with them until they completely fall asleep again.

In adults, night terrors can be triggered by stress, sleep deprivation or sleeping in a different bed. Studies have also shown that there is a higher incidence of night terrors among college students and those experiencing anxiety. Sleeping on your back also increases the likelihood of night terrors. They are typically treated with exercise, relaxation techniques and good sleep routine, although in severe cases medication may be needed.

WHAT YOUR DREAMS REALLY MEAN

There have long been many theories about the meanings of dreams. For example, Carl Jung's theory of the collective unconscious was that humans have a common store of inherited patterns of experiences and instincts, which are expressed in dreams in universal symbols he called archetypes. Today's psychologists, however, insist that dream symbols differ depending on the dreamer, and that the best person to interpret and understand your dream symbols is you.

You need to bear in mind that although dreams work in symbols and metaphors they are rarely literal. For one person a dream about a pizza may suggest a trip to Italy, and could be their subconscious urging them to take a break or holiday. For another, pizza could signify guilty feelings about breaking a diet.

Certain symbols, actions and colours in dreams can have universal interpretations. For example, pregnancy is often a symbol of new beginnings. Certain colours tend to represent particular emotions: red means action and desire; blue calmness and harmony; black is intimidating, and so on. However, one size can never fit all when it comes to dream interpretation. Every dreamer draws on their own personal experience to reflect their associations. One technique used by psychologists is the dream interview where people are asked a series of questions about their dreams in order to help them gain insight into their dreaming or unconscious mind.

HOW TO USE YOUR DREAMS

The images in your dreams are your own thoughts, images and feelings turned into a series of pictures. To better interpret them, try to make associations between your dreams and your current waking circumstances, thoughts and feelings. Bear in mind that people in your dreams can represent aspects of yourself. Can you detect any themes from the dream? Look for patterns over several dreams that might help explain an individual dream. And don't forget that not all dreams are deeply meaningful. Just as some movies are more compelling and thought-provoking than others, some dreams – like those when you are flying or surfing – are simply to be enjoyed.

SLEEP ON IT

The dreaming mind is more insightful than the waking mind, and it's long been known that people can solve problems by 'sleeping on it'. Some psychologists believe it is possible to take charge of your dreams so that they offer solutions to dilemmas in waking life. This is a process called dream incubation.

To incubate a dream you need to think about an issue or a problem you want your dream to resolve or a question you want answered. For example, should you apply for that job, move house or change career? During the day, write down your question on a piece of paper and read it over and over again. Keep it in your mind during the day, and just before you go to bed tell yourself that you will have the dream you want. Then leave your dream intention to incubate. Stop thinking about your intention to dream and let it go so that you can relax and calm your mind before you sleep.

LUCID DREAMING

Some researchers even believe that you can guide your dreams while you're sleeping. This process, called lucid dreaming, is when a sleeping person realises they are dreaming in the dream.

Lucid dreamers often turn their dreams into exciting fantasy adventures. They can travel in space and time, or holiday on an exotic beach with a celebrity, while being fully aware that they are dreaming. It is thought that lucid dreaming techniques can be used to solve problems, develop creative ideas, overcome fear and heal grief. For example, someone who is afraid of heights can climb Everest in their dream, and someone mourning the loss of a relative can meet them again in their dreams.

Lucid dreaming gives you the power to change the outcome of your dreams. Basically, you can do or be what you want, and that sense of empowerment and positive expectation can carry over into your waking life.

WHAT IF YOU CAN'T REMEMBER YOUR DREAMS?

Everybody dreams several times a night, and it has been estimated that we each have 100,000 dreams over the course of our lives. That's a whole lot of free therapy! So you might be wondering why you can't remember a single one. Medications, alcohol, stress and poor sleep routine can all block dream recall, so if you follow the sleep tips in this book you are far more likely to remember your dreams.

One way to ensure you remember your dreams is to tell yourself before you go to sleep that you will remember them on waking. You could even visualise yourself waking up in the morning and remembering your dreams. You are also more likely to remember your dreams if you keep a notebook or tape recorder by your bed and record them immediately on waking, even if that is in the middle of the night. Dreams fade very quickly from memory so it is crucial that you capture them as soon as you can. Don't wait till it's time to get up or after you brush your teeth. If you do that you will forget and lose a valuable dream.

Waking naturally without an alarm clock will also encourage dream recall, and if you follow the advice in this book an alarm clock should become unnecessary as your body and mind settle into a regular cycle of quality sleep. It also helps to wake up slowly. For a few moments when you wake up lie still with your eyes closed, as in some instances your dream may be related to the body position you lie in.

It may take days, or even weeks, before you're able to recall your dreams in detail, but keep trying. With practice, you will soon get into the habit of remembering and recording your dreams. Lucid dreaming, or being able to actually step into your dream and control the action while it is happening, may not be achievable for everyone but it is possible for everyone to recall their dreams and interpret the insightful messages they are sending.

Your dreams really are like a blockbuster movie where you are the writer, the director, the cameraman or woman, the star and the supporting cast. And what's now clear is that you are also the most discerning movie critic because the best person to understand and gain insight from your dreams is you.

Good Night!

As our understanding of the importance of sleep for peak performance and productivity becomes clearer, the issue of how to manage sleep in the context of our busy lives becomes ever more pressing.

In this 24/7 world we live in, the question of how little sleep we can get by on is the subject of much debate and research. There is no doubt that in the years to come the way we sleep will change; biofeedback techniques and drugs that can optimise brain power and minimise the time we need to spend asleep are already available.

Understanding the factors that affect sleep may soon lead to revolutionary new therapies for sleep disorders and to ways of overcoming jet lag and the problems associated with overtime. The benefits of napping are also being investigated. There is powerful evidence of their ability to boost memory, concentration and productivity at work. A number of enlightened companies have installed sleep pods – specially designed chairs for scheduled napping with visors to block out light and alarms – into 'wellness rooms'.

All the signs are that one day we may be able to eliminate our need to sleep altogether and throw away books like this. Is that a good thing? From a productivity point of view, possibly, but from a personal point of view, how many of us would really be willing to eliminate sleep completely?

How many of us would be willing to forgo the comfort of snuggling down in bed at night or that sleepy, dreamy feeling in the early morning when time stands still? How many of us could give up the wonderful feeling of someone you love falling asleep in your arms? And how many of us would miss our dreams – perhaps the only time we can become who and what we want and dwell in an utterly fantastic world of our own making?

Whatever direction sleep research takes, one thing is clear: sleep is an active and dynamic state that greatly influences our waking hours. To fully understand how the brain works and to optimise brain function we must understand sleep and maximise the quality of the sleep we get. More sleep research is needed. Given the fact that we spend more than a third of our lives asleep, it is high time we found out what was going on.

With a healthy sleep routine there is no doubt that your daytime potential for health, happiness, productivity and success is maximised. The sleeping brain is not a wasteland of inactivity but highly active. It performs numerous essential tasks from keeping us alive to enabling us to remember the past, seize the moment and imagine the future. I hope that after reading my guidelines in this book, getting a good night's sleep and feeling energetic, alert and productive every day will no longer be a sweet dream but an exciting reality.

TOP TIPS FOR A GOOD NIGHT'S SLEEP

You don't need to lie in: The sooner you understand that it is the quality of your sleep that counts rather than the quantity, the better. Just as too much food is unhealthy, so is too much sleep. So on days off don't indulge in a long lie-in thinking it's doing you the power of good. It's far healthier to get up when you wake up naturally.

Lights out: Sleep in complete darkness or as close as possible. Even a tiny bit of light in your room can disrupt your sleep rhythm and your pineal gland's production of sleep-inducing melatonin. There should also be as little light as possible in the bathroom if you get up in the middle of the night. As soon as you turn on that bright light you will for that night immediately cease production of the important sleep aid melatonin.

Avoid watching television and using the computer just before bed: Even better, get the television and laptop out of the bedroom completely. They can be too stimulating to the brain and disrupt the function of your pineal gland, which means it will take longer to fall asleep.

Stay cool: Keep the temperature in your bedroom no higher than 21°C (70°F). Many people keep their homes, and particularly the upstairs bedrooms, too hot.

Stay regular: You should go to bed, and wake up, at the same times each day, even at weekends. This will help your body to get into a sleep rhythm and make it easier to fall asleep and get up in the morning. Ideally, you should aim to be in bed before 11pm and to be up before 7.30am. Your body systems, particularly the adrenals, do the majority of their recharging or recovering during the hours of 11pm and 1am.

Keep active: At least 30 minutes of exercise every day, such as brisk walking, is recommended to help you drift off to sleep at night. Both your body and your mind need to have a workout during the day.

Consider buying a new bed: If your bed is more than eight years old, think about replacing it. Its structure will have deteriorated by up to 75 per cent, causing sleep disruption and potential damage to the spine. Research shows buying a new bed is more effective than sleeping pills and can improve a night's sleep by 42 minutes.

Use sunlight to set your biological clock: As soon as you get up in the morning, go outside and get some fresh air for 10 minutes. The bright sunlight (or any bright light) tells your body's natural biological clock that it's time to wake up, and that same clock will then be set to tell your body it's time to go to sleep about 14–16 hours later.

Pull your socks up: Wear socks to bed. Although your bedroom needs to stay cool, you won't get a good night's sleep if your feet are too cold. The feet often feel cold before the rest of the body due to their relatively poor circulation, and a study has shown that wearing socks reduces night waking.

Avoid alcohol and limit caffeine: Although alcohol makes people drowsy, the effect is short-lived and people will often wake up several hours later, unable to fall back to sleep. Alcohol will also keep you from falling into the deeper stages of sleep, where the body does most of its healing and recharging. Avoid drinking caffeine between three and eight hours before you need to sleep, depending on how sensitive you are to caffeine.

Establish a bedtime routine: This could include deep breathing, writing in a journal, reading or listening to relaxing music, having a warm bath with aromatherapy oils or indulging in a foot massage from your partner. Anything that clearly signals to your brain that it is bedtime is a good idea. The key is to find something that makes you feel relaxed and then repeat it each night to help you release the day's tensions and have the night of your dreams.

SLEEP CONTACTS

Sammy Margo
www.sammymargo.com
Tel: 020 7435 4910
E-mail: sleep@sammymargo.com
Sammy Margo is a chartered physiotherapist who is available for consultation.

The Chartered Society of Physiotherapy
www.csp.org.uk
Tel: 020 7306 6666
E-mail: enquiries@csp.org.uk
The Chartered Society of Physiotherapy (CSP) is the professional body for the UK's chartered physiotherapists, physiotherapy students and assistants.

British Snoring and Sleep Apnoea Association (BSSAA)
www.britishsnoring.co.uk
Tel: 01737 245638
E-mail: info@britishsnoring.co.uk
Offers help and support to those affected by snoring and sleep apnoea, information on causes and remedies and can provide anti-snoring and apnoea devices, including nasal sprays, mandibular advancement devices and nasal dilators.

The Sleep Council
www.sleepcouncil.com
Tel: 0845 0584595
E-mail: info@sleepcouncil.com
Promotes the benefits of sleeping well. Provides information leaflets on sleep and beds.

Sleep Apnoea Trust

www.sleep-apnoea-trust.org
Tel: 0845 6060685
E-mail: info@sleep-apnoea-trust.org
Provides information and support for sufferers and their families.

Narcolepsy Association UK (UKAN)

www.narcolepsy.org.uk
Tel: 0845 4500 394
E-mail: info@narcolepsy.org.uk
Promotes the interests of people with narcolepsy and encourages better understanding of the illness.

American Sleep Apnea Association

www.sleepapnea.org
E-mail: asaa@sleepapnea.org
A non-profit organisation dedicated to educating the public about sleep apnoea.

National Sleep Foundation

www.sleepfoundation.org
E-mail: nsf@sleepfoundation.org
American website with information on sleep and sleep disorders.

Sleep Disorder Clinics

Referral should be made through your GP.

Index